Smart and Pervasive Healthcare

Edited by Urvashi Sharma

Published in London, United Kingdom

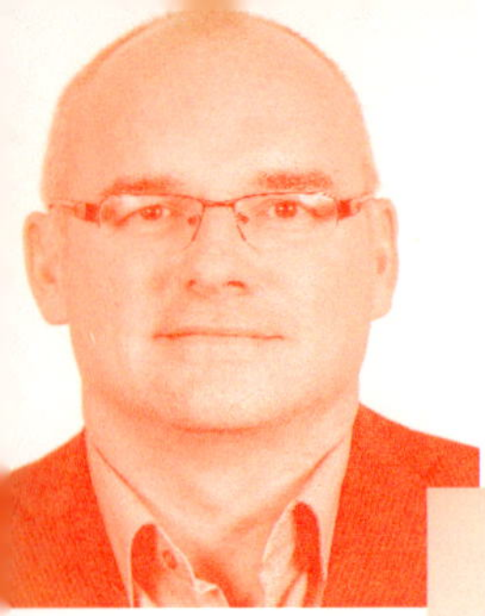
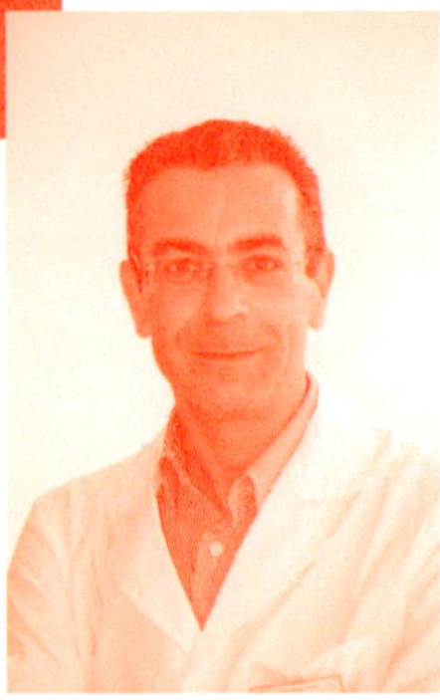
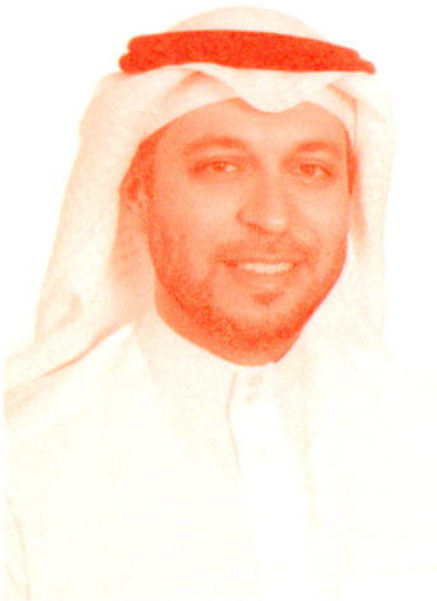
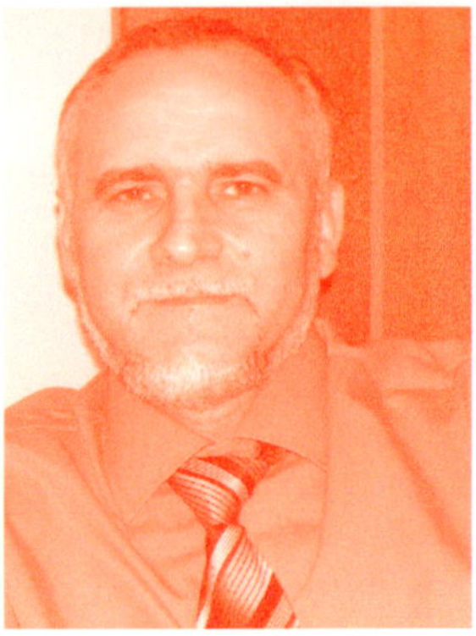
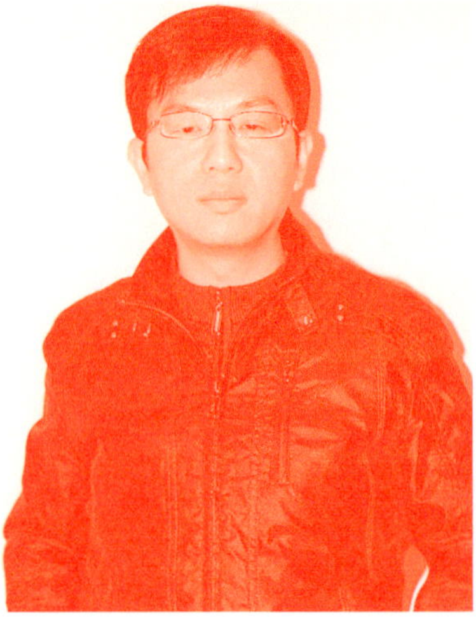
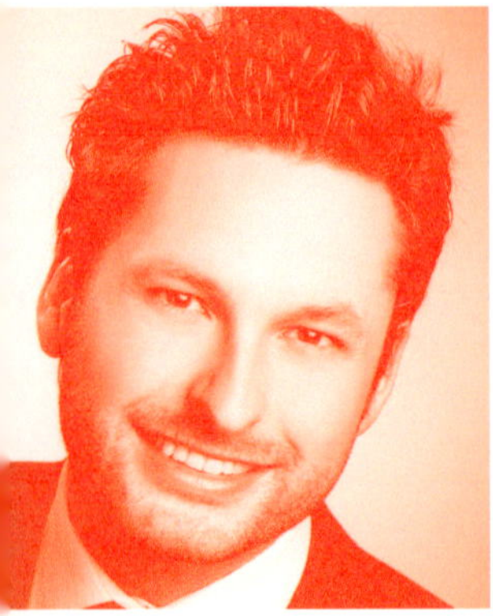
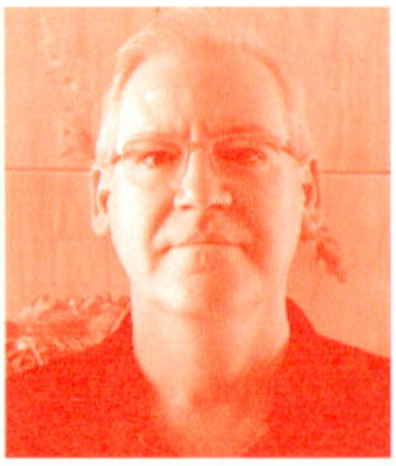

IntechOpen

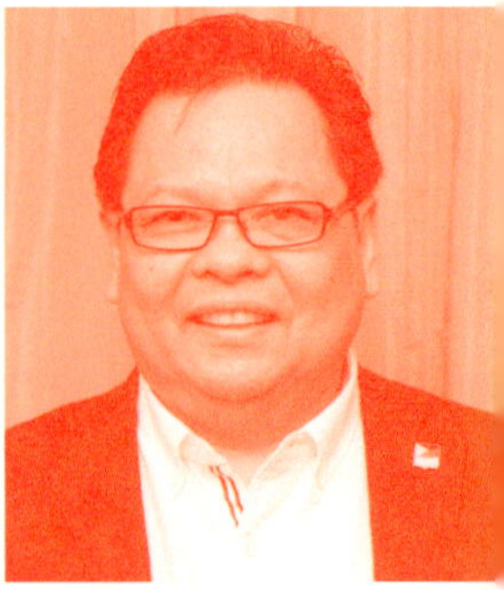
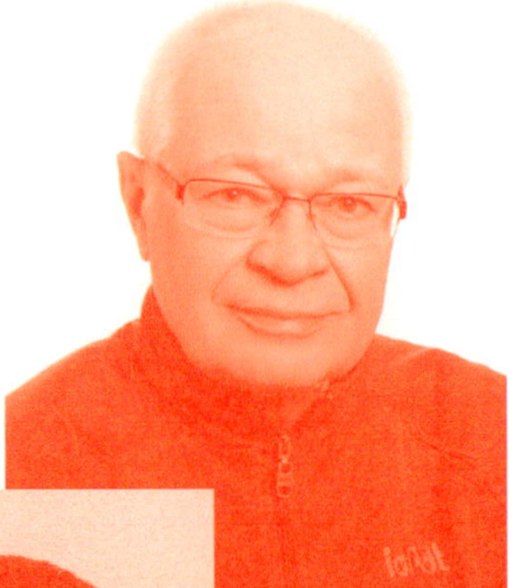
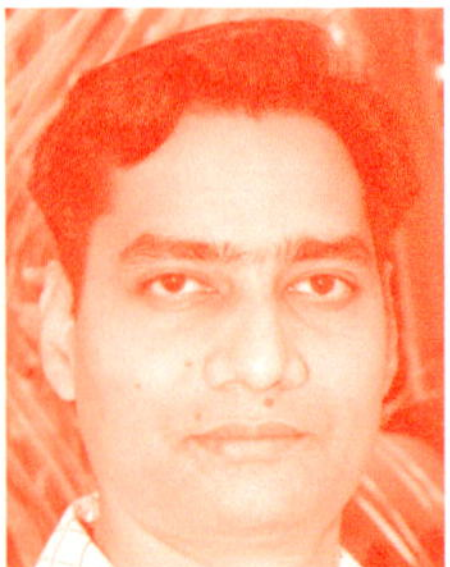
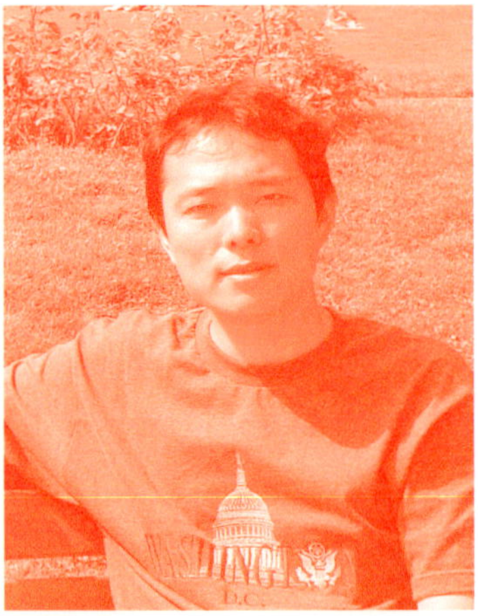
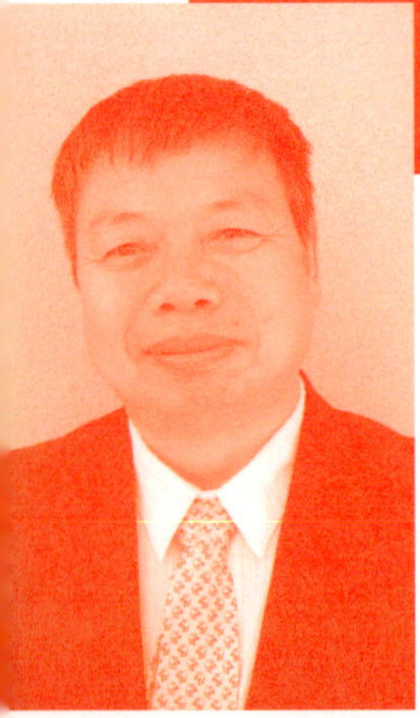
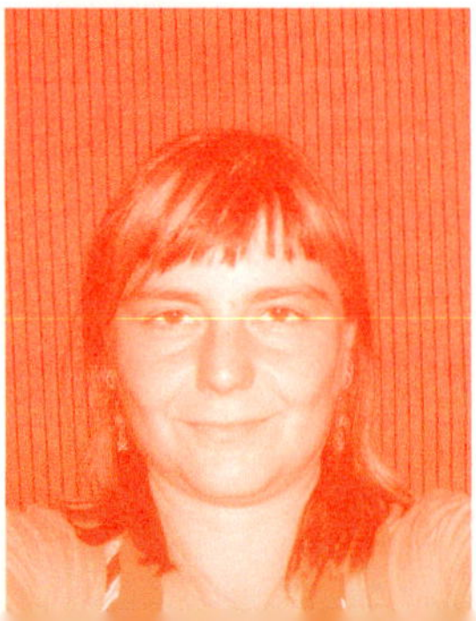

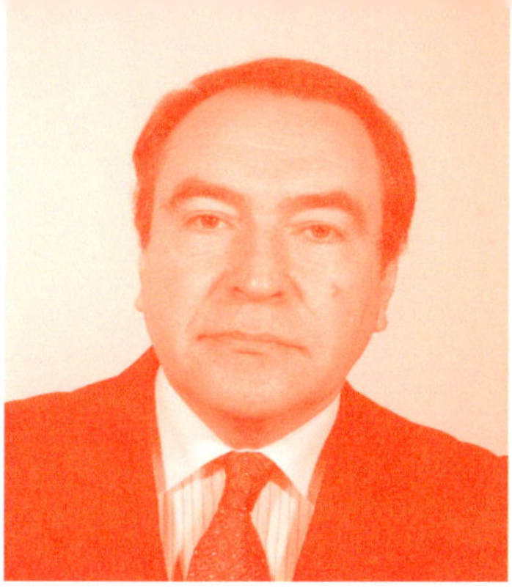
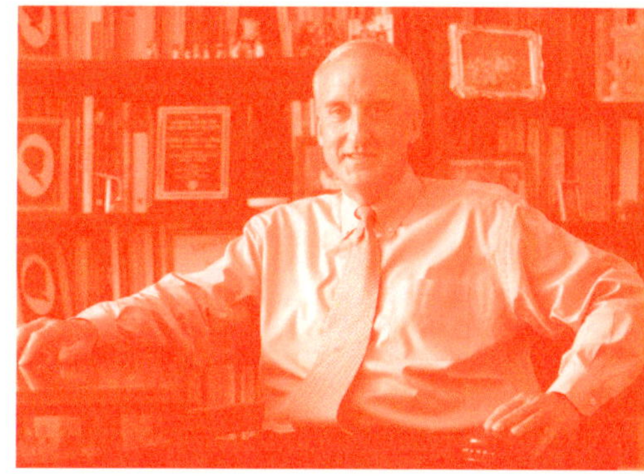
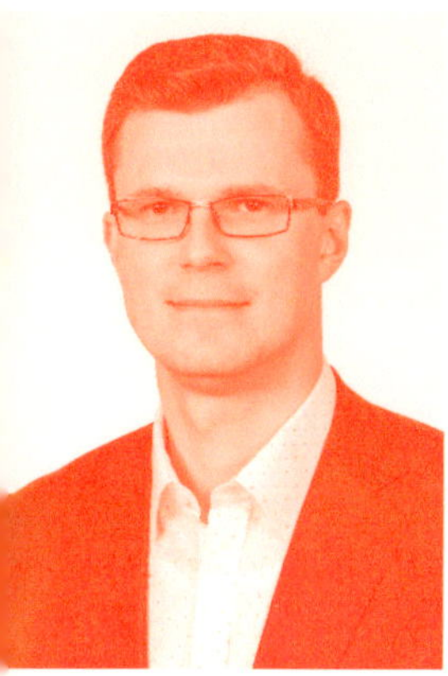
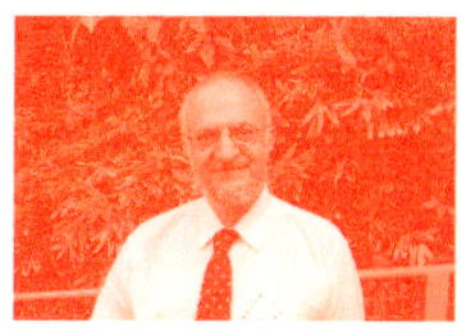
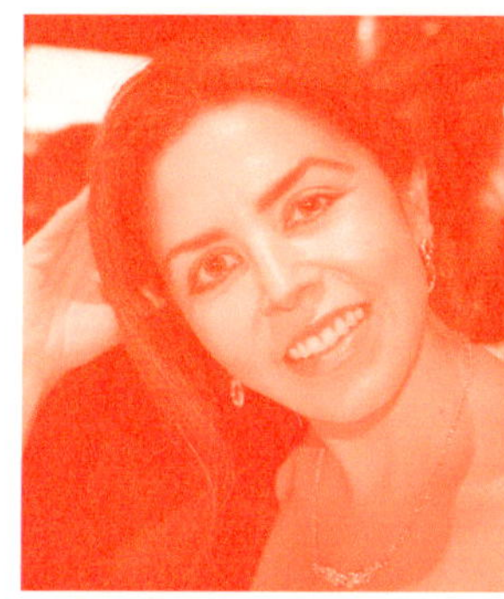

Supporting open minds since 2005

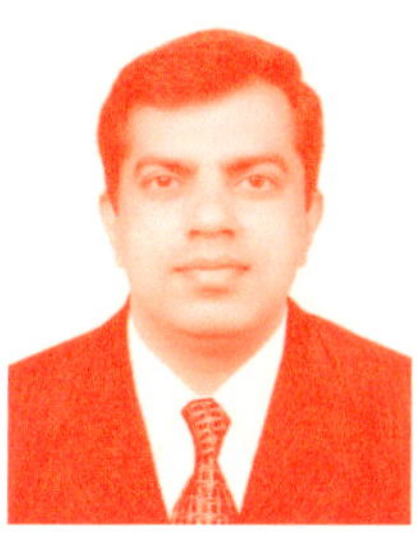
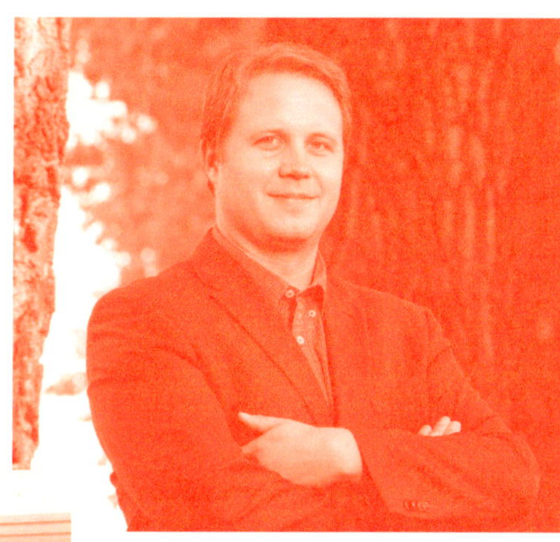
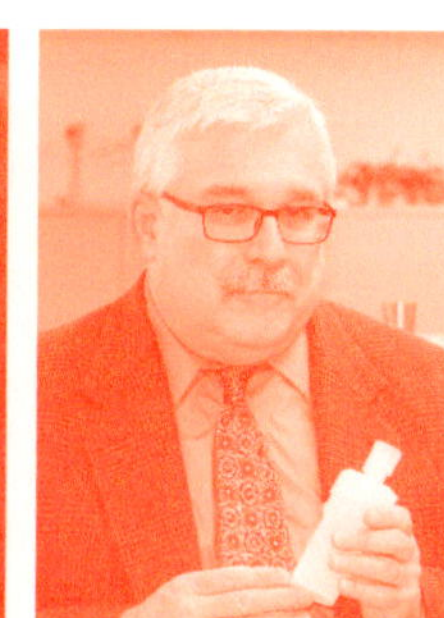
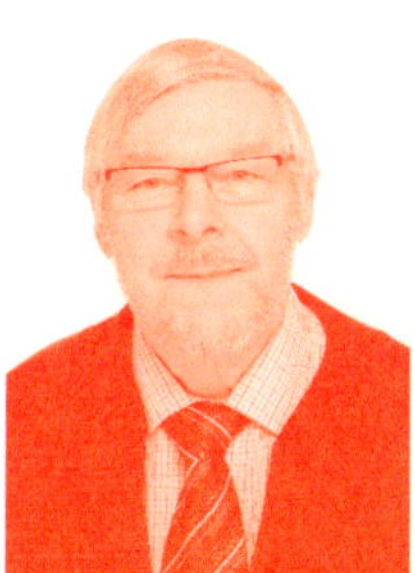
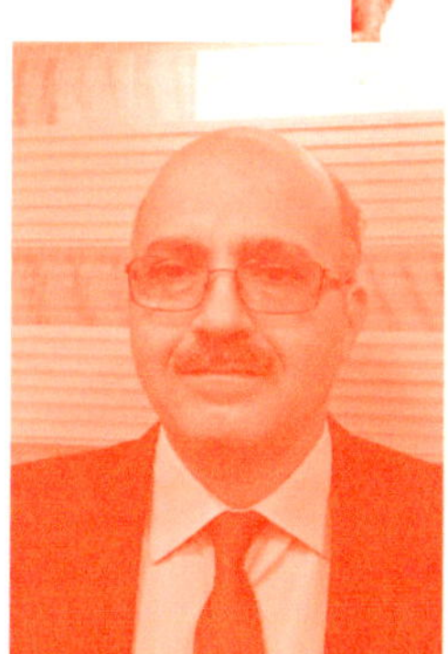
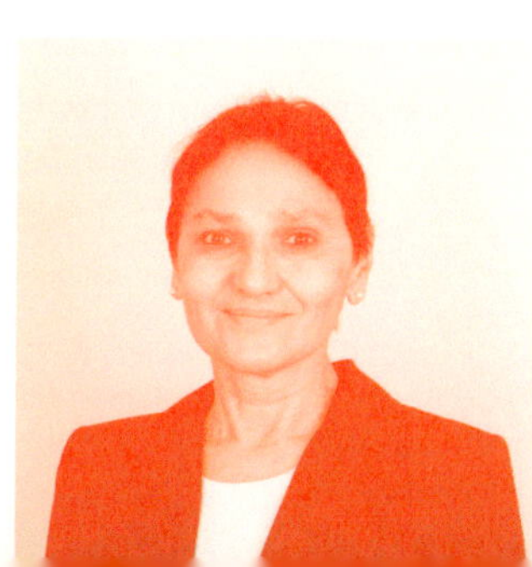
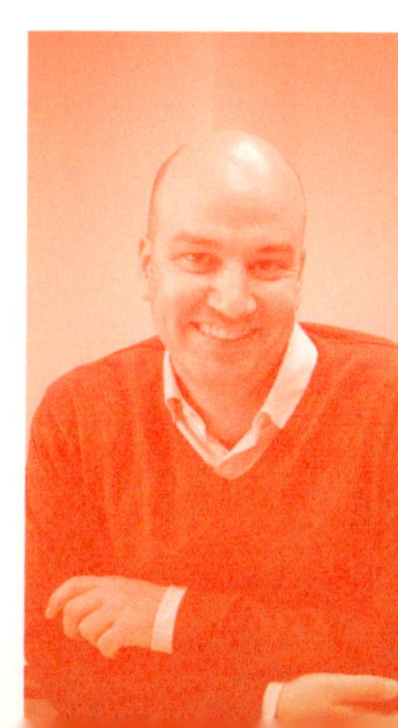

Smart and Pervasive Healthcare
http://dx.doi.org/10.5772/intechopen.91484
Edited by Urvashi Sharma

Contributors
Sofia Voutsidou, Eloisa Vargiu, Meritxell Gómez-Martínez, Laura Ros-Freixedes, Silvia Orte, Kian Seif, Felip Miralles, David Marí, Lo Fu Tan, Yu Liang, Dalei Wu, Zibin- Guo, Dakila Ledesma, Erkan Kaplanoglu, Anthony Skjellum, Karim Keshavejee, Dustin Johnston-Jewell, Brian Lee, Robert Kyba, Malcolm Clarke

First published in London, United Kingdom, 2022 by IntechOpen
IntechOpen is the global imprint of INTECHOPEN LIMITED, registered in England and Wales, registration number: 11086078, 5 Princes Gate Court, London, SW7 2QJ, United Kingdom
Printed in Croatia

British Library Cataloguing-in-Publication Data
A catalogue record for this book is available from the British Library

Additional hard and PDF copies can be obtained from orders@intechopen.com

Smart and Pervasive Healthcare
Edited by Urvashi Sharma
p. cm.
Print ISBN 978-1-83968-680-1
Online ISBN 978-1-83968-681-8
eBook (PDF) ISBN 978-1-83968-682-5

For EU product safety concerns:
IN TECH d.o.o., Prolaz Marije Krucifikse Kozulić 3, 51000 Rijeka, Croatia, info@intechopen.com or visit our website at intechopen.com.

Meet the editor

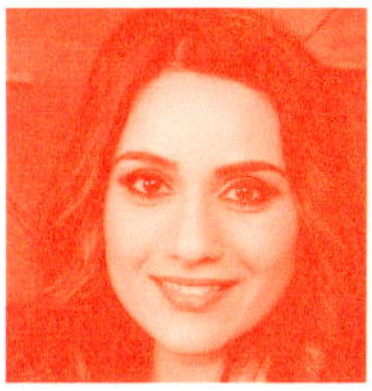

Dr. Urvashi Sharma has a BEng in Electronic and Electrical Engineering, MSc in Biomedical Engineering, MSc in Counselling and Psychotherapy, and Ph.D. in Healthcare Information Systems. She is driven by her passion to understand how human beings relate to and encounter interventions and innovations within a given context. Over the last seventeen years, Dr. Sharma has worked in different fields and sectors including education as well as health and social care. Her work has contributed to understanding the role of users and their context in relation to a successful application and use of interventions and/or innovations. She is a proponent of stakeholder engagement and involvement in decision making, and the application of appropriate research methodologies that enable exploration of lived experiences and provide deeper insights into what really matters to users.

Contents

Preface

Smart and pervasive healthcare aims at facilitating better healthcare access, provision, and delivery by overcoming spatial and temporal barriers. It provides opportunities to deliver healthcare solutions within complex and restrictive contexts, requiring input from different stakeholders and under demanding circumstances where traditional methods may not be adequate.

More importantly, with the COVID-19 pandemic requiring scientists, researchers, and healthcare providers around the world to rethink access to timely and effective health care and its delivery, the role that smart and pervasive healthcare can play is of growing interest.

This book provides valuable insights into how researchers across the globe are thinking about, working with, and furthering the boundaries of application and use of smart and pervasive healthcare-based solutions.

The content in this book will benefit anyone who is looking to find a way in which future healthcare access and delivery can be better shaped and benefited.

Dr. Urvashi Sharma
King's College London,
United Kingdom

Section 1

Remote Patient Monitoring

Chapter 1

Results from Telehealth

Malcolm Clarke

Abstract

Telemedicine and telehealth have a wide range of definitions and understanding. Telehealth has been described as taking many forms and having many terms to describe its activities such as; home health care, telecare, tele-dermatology, tele-psychiatry, tele-radiology, telemonitoring, and remote patient monitoring. In general, the purpose of telehealth is to acquire information on a patient in one location, make that information available in a separate location, usually for the convenience of the clinician, and then use that information to provide management to a patient, who may be in a further location, through the mediation of a remote clinician, or directly to the patient. Typically this has taken the form of the patient being in their own home or at a clinical establishment remote from the hospital such as the district hospital, remote clinic, and primary care, with clinical information being collected and transferred using technology between locations. This chapter focuses on results from telehealth in the form of remote patient monitoring (RPM), in which data is collected from the patient whilst they are in their own home, or other non-clinical setting such as residential care.

Keywords: telehealth results, telehealth outcomes, remote patient monitoring, RPM, cost-effectiveness, patient benefits, telehealth technology

1. Introduction

The earliest form of telehealth was via telephone, which has included patient-doctor consultation, doctor-doctor (specialist) for advice and referral, and clinician (nurse) led structured telephone support, with the first reports of management of chronic disease appearing in 1995 [1]. This review [1] shows a steady increase in the number of reports from telehealth from 1995 to 2011 (**Figure 1**), with the greater number of reports being on management of diabetes, followed by congestive heart failure (CHF) and chronic obstructive pulmonary disease (COPD), with smaller numbers for asthma and hypertension. There has been continued growth and the Covid pandemic of 2020 has caused significant increase in its use.

Telehealth has mainly been favoured in locations where significant distance between parties is involved, such as between primary and secondary/tertiary care, with most of the results being reported from countries such as USA and Australia, where significant distance between sites is involved. In a review [2], more than 50% of reported results were from USA.

Telehealth has been applied in many applications. **Figure 2** shows the range identified in a review of reported successes and failures [3], together with the perceived advantages that were provided in the studies in **Figure 3**.

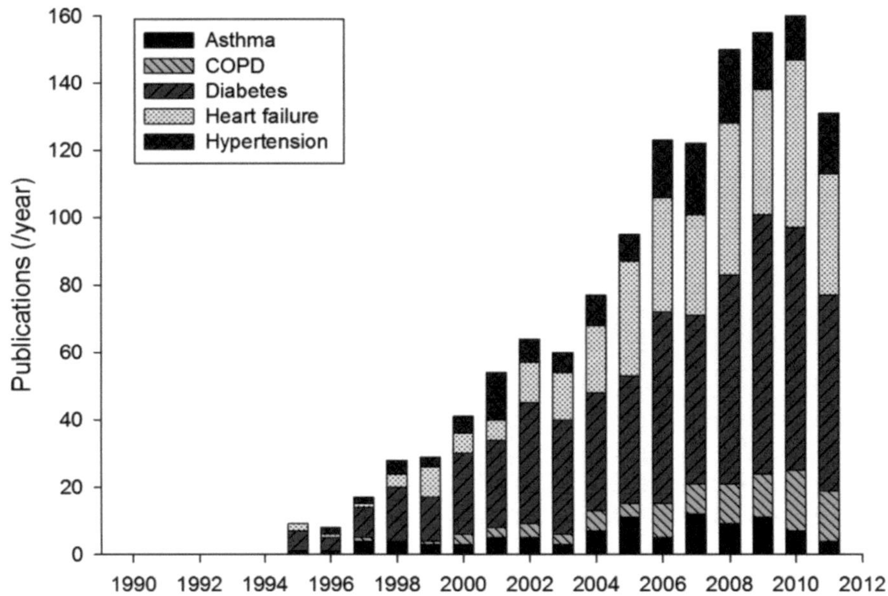

Figure 1.
Telehealth publications by year [1].

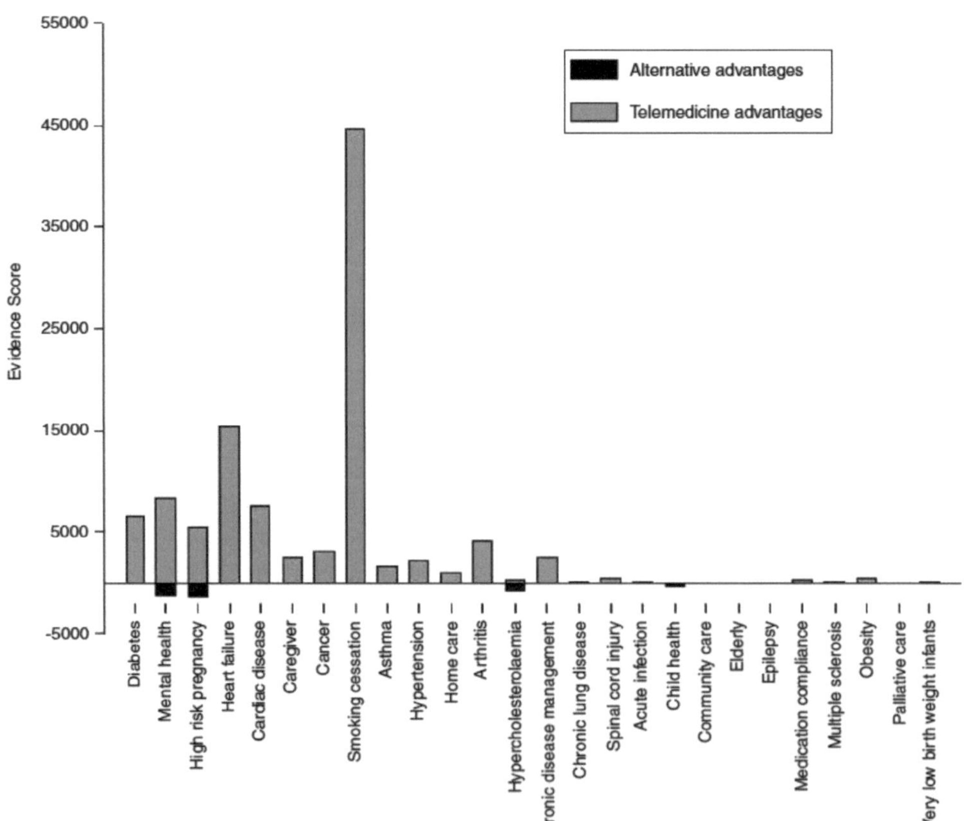

Figure 2.
Advantages of telehealth by application [3].

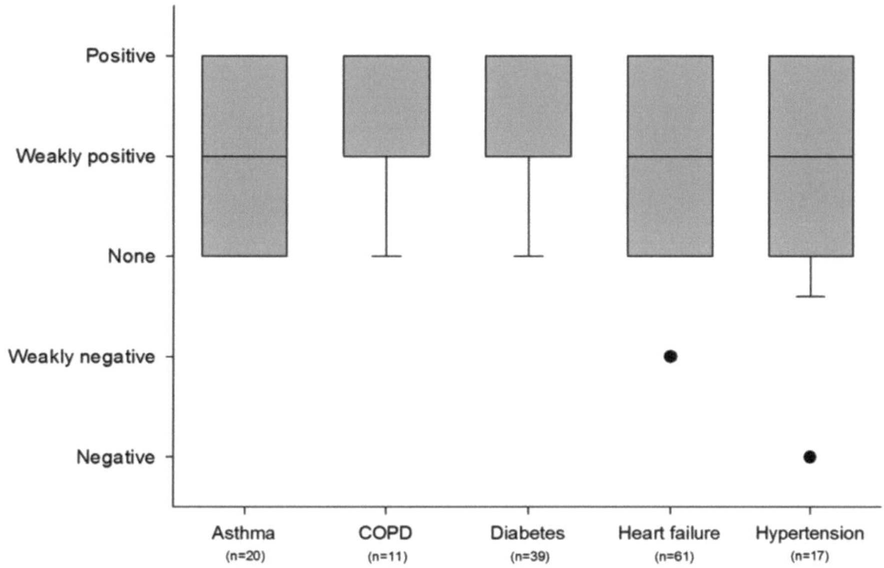

Figure 3.
Advantages of Telehealth by application [3].

However the application of telehealth remains intermittent and patchy and its use has been determined primarily where economic advantage can be demonstrated. This is most frequently demonstrated where the economic benefits of introduction can be gained elsewhere within the same organisation through savings in travel or impact on the provision of services across the organisation. This is most clearly seen in the introduction of telehealth in the indigenous health programs in the USA, such as in Indian Health Service (IHS) providing services to reservations and the Alaska Federal Health Care Access Network (AFHCAN) providing services to remote Inuit communities [4]. These have exploited store-and-forward telehealth to support services such as diabetic retinopathy (IHS), and a wide range of services including ENT, dermatology, and ECG examinations (AFHCAN), for which a purpose cart was designed.

The Veterans Administration (VA) is a US Federal programme that provides health care to those who have served in any of the US armed forces and their families, whilst in the forces and upon discharge anywhere within the US. Many of retired return or settle in small communities throughout the US, which may be far from VA clinical facilities. In order to serve these patients, the VA instigated a programme of telehealth that included many approaches that included video clinic telehealth and store-and-forward being used for home monitoring and capturing retinal images to manage diabetic retinopathy. The use of the programme between 1994 and 2014 is reported in [5] and the increasing number of encounters using the store-and-forward is shown in **Figure 4**.

The growth in use of telehealth within the VA continues, with the latest release of a request for procurement in 2021 for over $1 billion, accelerated in response to the Covid pandemic, with most patients preferring to consult with their doctor from home [6].

There are similar experiences of an increase in the use of telehealth during the Covid pandemic. For example the NHS in the UK turned to online and telephone consultations with GPs (family doctor). It is to be seen how delivery of health will evolve post Covid.

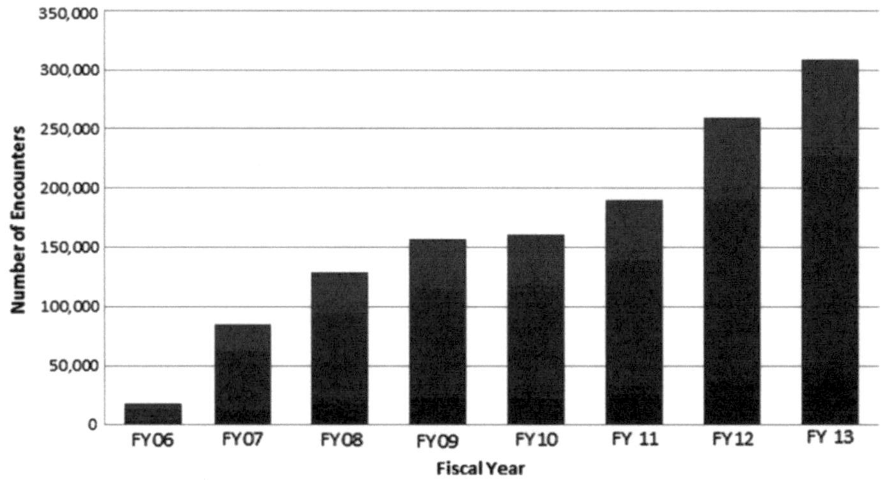

Figure 4.
Veterans Health Affairs store-and-forward telehealth encounters, fiscal years 2006–2013 [5].

2. Acceptance and feasibility

The majority of the projects undertaken to evaluate telehealth have been small scale pilots that include only small numbers of patients and run for relatively short periods, reporting short-term outcomes. This presents difficulty in determining the effect of telehealth on clinical outcomes and obtaining evidence on other benefits such as economic outcome. For this reason such projects generally report on measurable outcomes that include feasibility and acceptance of the technology by the users; patient and/or clinician, with the majority of studies on the clinicians. Despite the limited outcome of such studies, they can provide valuable information on understanding how technology should be introduced to promote successful adoption, and data to direct larger studies.

Most studies on acceptance are based on one of the models of user acceptance, with the Technology Acceptance Model (TAM) [7, 8] being particularly popular, which considers perceived usefulness and ease of use to be its primary constructs. However this approach has limitations when applied to evaluation of telehealth.

2.1 Acceptance by the clinician

A systematic review [9] on factors affecting front-line staff acceptance of telehealth technologies identified the factors that can act as facilitators (**Table 1**) or barriers (**Table 2**), and their importance.

A further systematic review of the experiences of nursing professionals [10] reinforced the findings of [9] and expanded detail on some of the topics to include aspects such as prior experience with technology. It also focussed on the post-experience of telehealth rather than prospective perspectives of participants and recognised that, although the nature and practice of delivering care may have changed during the project, this brought advantages, such as the ability to monitor more parameters and provided a continuous flow of information.

Longitudinal studies such as [11] are therefore invaluable in identifying the preconceptions of the users and understanding how these might change during the course of usage of the technology. Such studies also show how certain personality types will remain resistant and seek to influence the group dynamic to thwart the

Facilitators to staff acceptance	Occurrence
Easy-to-use, reliable equipment	7
Collaboration	6
Training and support	5
Flexible and responsive working practices	4
Risk and safety assessment	4
Integration into routine practice	3
Personalization and patient feedback	3
Strong leadership and local champions	3
Trust in technology and service design	3
Maintaining quality of staff–patient interactions	2

Table 1.
Facilitators to staff acceptance [9].

Barriers to staff acceptance	Occurrence
Negative impact of service change/implementation	7
Negative impact on staff–patient relationship	7
Low expectations of outcomes/need	6
Negative impact on staff autonomy/credibility	6
Interoperability, information sharing and data security	5
Technical/usage issues	5
Concerns about user-friendliness	4
Reliability/accuracy concerns	4
Technophobia/lack of confidence in technology	4
Installation issues	3
No reduction in workload/improvements in efficiency	3
Patient safety concerns	3
Poor change management	3
Communication issues	2
Lack of training	2

Table 2.
Barriers to staff acceptance [9].

introduction of new technology and approaches. Such insight is essential to understand effective techniques for change management.

The standard approach in information systems research is to understand the dynamics of interaction between the key stakeholders, the wider context of the organisation, external factors, and the technology innovation, through models and frameworks. The usual technique is based on grounded theory, where information is gathered through interviews, communications and documentation, and analysed to determine the themes (often by frequency analysis) that are then connected together.

A general view of this approach may be seen in the Triality Framework [12], which relates all possible interactions between the key stakeholders (the technology, the organisation, and the user), highlighting how the interactions may include a two-way effect, which extends significantly the concepts which should be considered compared to TAM (**Figure 5**).

Therefore a broader consideration of interaction will bring in the concepts of the Triality Framework [12], and that are highlighted within the factors of **Table 1** and **Table 2**, such as acceptability (does it provide for the role of users), demand (are changes required), efficacy (does it fulfill the role), expertise (are users able to use the technology), trust (is it reliable and safe), legitimacy (does it meet legal requirements), optimality (does it perform the task), and equity (does it provide equal service to all patients).

2.2 Acceptance by the patient

Patient acceptance is less well studied and understood as it is influenced by very many more factors than acceptance by the clinician. However the majority of the studies using TAM have been conducted in the work place on cohorts largely familiar with technology. Patients present very different characteristics and circumstances and therefore have different motivations and responses.

For example, one study [13] used assessment of the perceived usefulness of telehealth services to act as a predictor of acceptance, but had to extend the concepts to include effort expectancy, social influence, and facilitating conditions as its root constructs when applied to patients.

Moreover it is essential not to consider patients as a homogeneous group; patients differ greatly by age, education, social status, economic status, belief, coping strategy, stage of disease, prior experience, familiarity with technology,

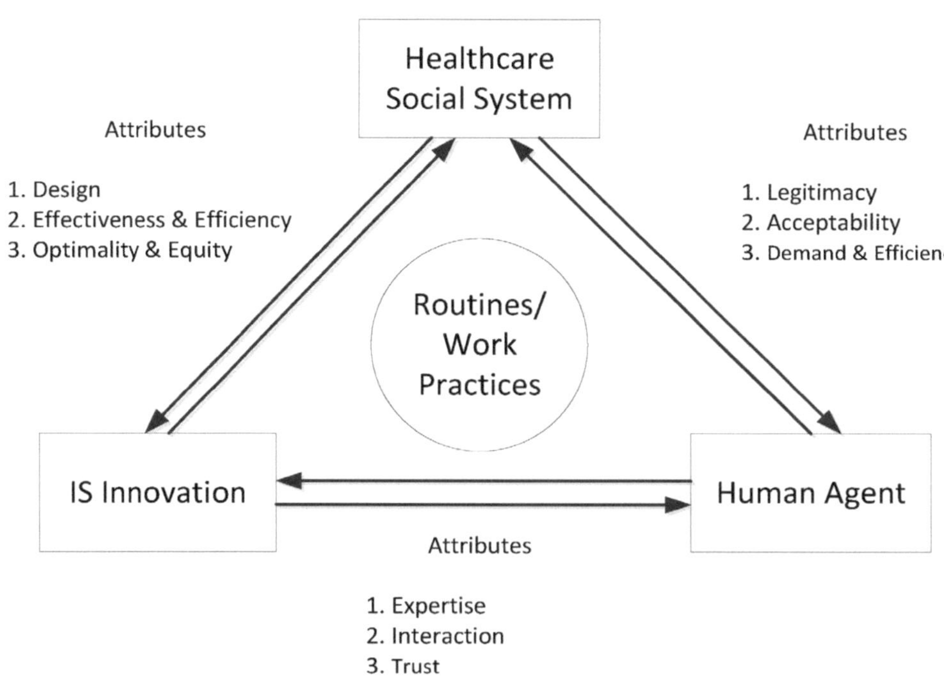

Figure 5.
Triality framework [12].

surrounding support, relationship with their physician, and location. A much richer model to describe factors affecting patient technology acceptance is required.

In one model [14], age and stage of illness are considered as primary influences, and further recognises that age impacts illness and that the severity of illness can impact on the age perceived by the patient. The patient then brings a further multiplicity of factors that affects their willingness to accept telehealth and continue its use.

In addition, the approach and support of the physician can influence the understanding of the need and purpose for telehealth, and thus the acceptance and use (**Figure 6**).

The effect of the stage of illness is considered in the transtheoretical model (TTM) [15] which identifies individuals moving through six stages as their condition changes:

- Pre-contemplation stage - not thinking about their health condition, or ready to change their behaviour related to the problem.

- Contemplation stage - begin to recognize their health problem and consider the pros and cons of seeking treatment.

- Preparation stage - intention to take action and may make small behaviour changes.

- Action stage - take overt steps to treat their health condition.

- Maintenance stage - able to sustain the health changes they have made.

- Termination – added by some to complete the stages.

It is observed that people in the later stages of the TTM are more likely to pursue intervention and are more likely to have successful outcomes than people in earlier stages, and therefore adhere to a programme of telehealth.

Age has a major influence on acceptance of a technological approach. For example, a survey of usage of smartphones [14] reveals the majority of people over 60 are

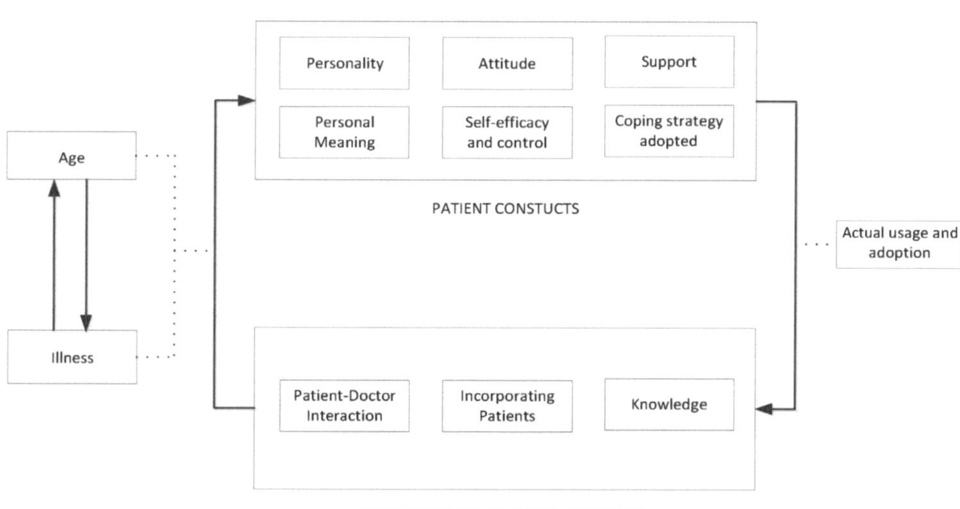

Figure 6.
Patient Technology Acceptance Model (PTAM) [14].

non-users (with many others having only trivial use), with a significant proportion of people in the 46-59 age group also being non-uses. A similar proportion will not have access to broadband, and many will have little or no experience of use of technology. It is therefore important to understand how to deploy telehealth in a non-threatening and unobtrusive way. It is therefore appropriate to develop specific models to describe the behaviour of the elderly, such as the Senior Patient Technology Model [16], that must address the specific concerns of this group, such as stigmatisation, simplicity, unobtrusive, independent (no reliance on broadband or telephone), non-threatening, and privacy in use (hidden from general view). It should complement their relationship with the clinician, and not threaten to remove (**Figure** 7).

2.3 Factors for readiness and adoption

In addition to consideration of the acceptance by the patient and the clinician, there is also a need to understand the readiness of an organisation to host telehealth. This can include understanding the readiness of the technology and the key stakeholders.

Readiness of technology will include understanding the availability and capability of the communication technology (networks) that will span between the parties involved in the telehealth activity, and the availability of suitable end equipment. Understanding the availability and capability of the technology can be complex, as this must be assessed for its ability to support specific applications; the bandwidth and delay required for video and store-and-forward are quite different and will be affected in different ways. Likewise the bandwidth required to transfer images and a vital sign will be quite different. Network capability can easily be assessed by consideration of the technology being used, undertaking performance measurements on the network using one of the many tools such as iPerf [17], and assessing the performance of typical applications. For example, in the implementation of the AFHCAN network, the large delays experienced using a satellite based network caused problems in many applications that were based on the TCP protocol (such as web), and had to be modified to use the UDP protocol.

Assessing readiness of the key stakeholders takes the form administering questionnaires (quantitative research) and conducting interviews through focus groups

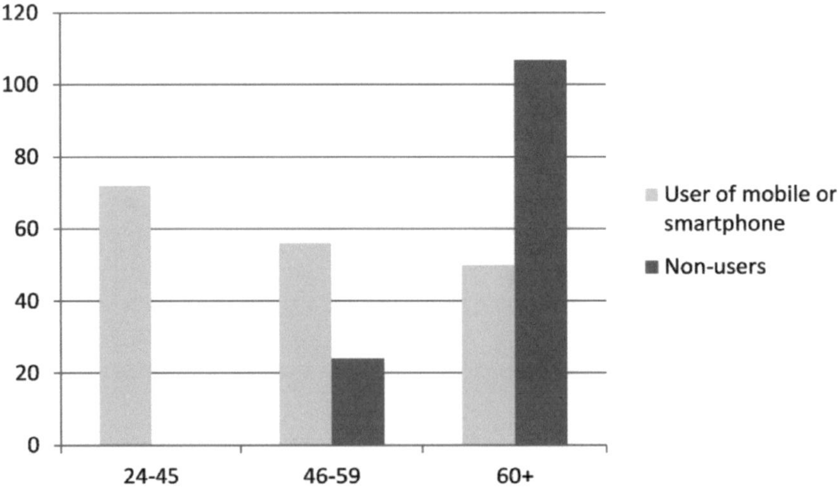

Figure 7.
Smartphone Usage [14].

and with individuals to gain deeper understanding (qualitative research) (see [18] for details on design of research studies).

Issues that are raised can be complex depending on the country, politics and situation, and may not relate only to professional issues. For example [19] considers the effects of culture on the acceptance of telehealth in Middle Eastern countries. Standardized methodology has been developed in order to undertake assessment of readiness in studies such [20].

2.4 Feasibility and acceptance

Most projects that develop or investigate use of technology will report on its feasibility and acceptance. Such projects tend to include small numbers of patients, are short duration, and study a single group. There is also a tendency for projects to be repetitive of earlier work. Outcomes are therefore limited in scope. However they can provide anecdotal evidence to guide design and small scale results that can be used in the design of larger trials. These projects have a tendency to be over-zealous in their approach to evaluation. For example [21] references 10 similar pilot studies and administered a questionnaire with 37 questions to patients. The project also found that 84% of the participants preferred the telehealth to having to visit the hospital and 87% were very or extremely satisfied. This is a common outcome in such short term projects.

However the reasons for the acceptance may need to be fully understood in order to interpret outcome appropriately. In [21] patients with postpartum hypertension were monitored at home, in place of having to travel to hospital with a new-born, waiting in an out-patient clinic with a fractious baby, and interfering with feeding and sleep. However this small study also reported that 16% of participants developed severe hypertension, 45% had some change of medication and 11% had to be referred to the emergency department for evaluation of symptomatic severe hypertension. None were referred for readmission. Such data can inform likely group size in larger studies and determine prevalence in outcomes if deployed at scale.

3. Types of technology

3.1 Vital signs sensors

Many devices have been developed and employed for telehealth:

- Blood pressure meter – CHF, diabetes, hypertension, pre-eclampsia
- Weigh scale - CHF
- Pulse oximeter - COPD
- Glucose meter – diabetes
- Peak flow meter – asthma
- ECG – coronary artery disease, arrhythmia, atrial fibrillation
- Body composition analyser – CHF
- Thermometer - infection

- Insulin pump – managing diabetes
- Urine analysis – self-testing urine infection and presence of other conditions
- Sleep apnoea breathing therapy equipment (SABTE) – home management of sleep apnoea
- Continuous glucose monitor - diabetes
- Spirometer - COPD
- INR – anti-coagulation therapy

Each of these devices has an IEEE 11073 standard to define communication of its data. Several of these devices are available based on Blue Tooth Low Energy as wireless connection, although the data format is generally proprietary. Some devices follow the respective Blue Tooth device profile.

3.2 Assisted living

Telehealth for assisted living can be used to support people in their own home (referred as telecare) and can complement monitoring vital signs. Many forms of sensor are possible, from simple emergency buttons and pull-cords activated by the occupant (personal emergency response sensor - PERS), fall sensors, and sensors that monitor the environment of the occupant. Simple environmental sensors can

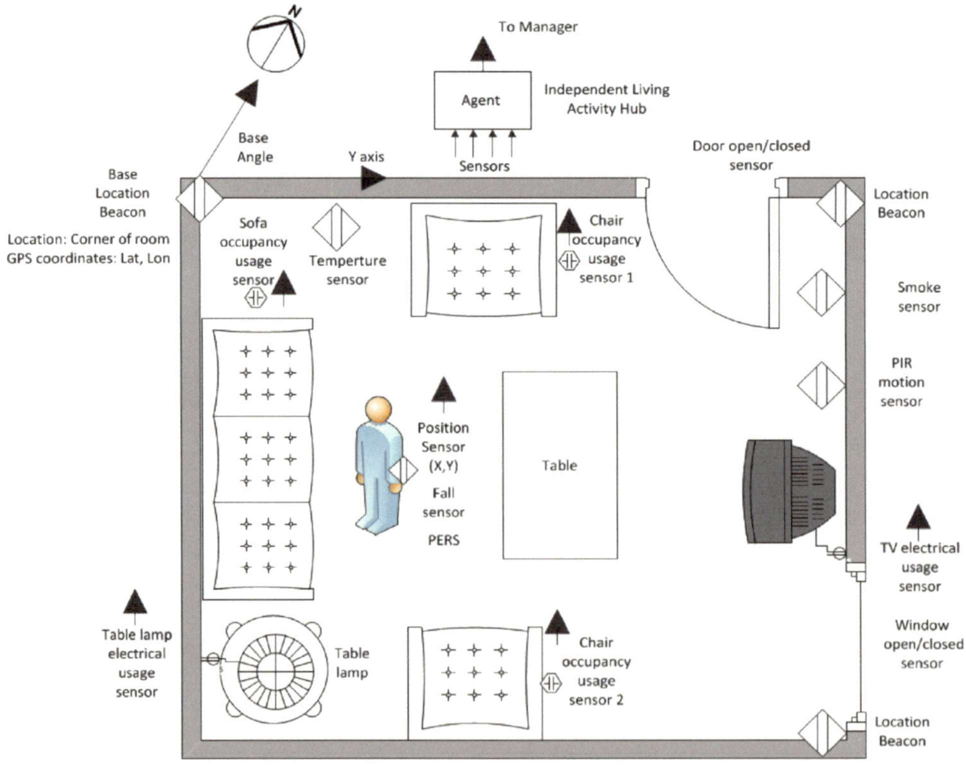

Figure 8.
Assisted Living Sensors (IEEE 11073-10471).

generate alerts such as for high or low temperature. Others sensors can monitor activity, such as use of appliances, room occupancy, or occupancy of bed/chair, from which behaviour might be inferred and alerts generated when there is departure.

Figure 8 shows the range of devices that could be deployed in an assisted living setting (taken from draft of IEEE 11073-10471) that provides a standard for transmission of data that is interoperable with the IEEE 11073-20601 [22] standard for vital signs sensors.

4. Patient benefits

4.1 Determining clinical benefits

The recognised approach to determine the effectiveness of any intervention is the randomised controlled trial (RCT), in which patients are randomly placed into groups that are designed to have equal statistics other than the intervention under study. This typically involves ensuring that each group has equal statistics for factors such as age, sex, and stage of disease. The best approach is to ensure that the type of intervention being administered is hidden from both the patient and the doctor, in the "double-blind RCT", with the patients receiving either the intervention or placebo in order to ensure they are unaware of the intervention and exclude other factors that might influence the outcome. This approach is often referred as the "gold standard" to determine outcome (see [18]) for details on design of research studies).

However evaluating technology presents difficulties as it is not easy to "hide" the use of technology from patients to implement a double-blind RCT. Alternative approaches are adopted. This usually takes one of two forms: comparing the results from large groups with and without the technology; or comparing the results of each patient with their own data before and after the introduction of the technology, sometimes referred as a "crossover" study. In the first approach, care must be taken to ensure sufficiently large groups for comparison so that they have otherwise matched statistics. The second approach requires care that results are not affected by the deterioration in the condition of the patient over the period of the research, and that seasonal effects on a disease such as flu in the autumn and any other influences of time on a disease are avoided.

The choice of which clinical benefits are assessed also presents difficulties as telehealth is not a treatment, therefore there is no direct outcome that can be measured; rather telehealth impacts diagnosis, decision, and management, and therefore impacts secondary outcomes. In addition, the design of the services that respond to the information collected from telehealth are as important as the design of the telehealth technology; and the intervention must be designed as a complete service, with consideration of the clinical services involved and the communication and relationship between the separate key stakeholders. This important aspect of design of a study is rarely discussed in reports, which not only prevents full comparison of method to be made, but does not allow full advantage of the experience to be gained.

The ultimate analysis of the outcome of assessment of clinical benefit is the systematic review and meta-analysis of outcomes, as these permit rigorous statistical evaluation of benefits of using telehealth over usual care from aggregation of the results from multiple studies. The systematic review has a specific methodology that defines how terms are used to identify trials and how the trials are selected for inclusion and exclusion based on factors such as the number in the trial, duration of the trial, and whether RCT [23]. A systematic review will normally use at least two reviewers to undertake the selection of papers, with an arbiter to make a final decision on selection. Outcomes from the selected trials may then be summarized and are frequently presented as a funnel plot (also referred as Forest plot) that shows the risk ratio of each study included in the analysis and overall outcome.

4.2 Assessing clinical outcome

The most common approach that is used to assess clinical outcome is through the use of a validated disease specific questionnaire. This assesses the perceived state of health of a patient and the perceived level of symptoms and their impact on everyday activities. Many such questionnaires exist for diseases such as CHF [24], COPD [25], and asthma [26].

The second approach is to use a questionnaire such as the EQ5D [27] or SF36 [28] to assess the perceived general state of health of a patient. Whilst use of these questionnaires does not assess clinical outcome directly, it can determine the perceived benefits the patient may feel from being monitored.

Direct assessment of clinical outcome is determined through disease specific measures such as ejection fraction in CHF, lung function in COPD, and glucose and HbA1c in diabetes. Secondary measures may be considered such as blood pressure in diabetes. Some projects assess secondary outcomes that include death rate, and extension of life.

4.3 Clinical benefits in patients with CHF

CHF is a common chronic condition with a prevalence of about 13% amongst those aged 85 years or above in countries such as the UK [29]. Telehealth in CHF has been found to improve health outcome for patients and reduce the number of hospitalisations [30, 31]. Many studies have considered nurse telephone support and remote patient monitoring as equivalent and either report combined outcomes or present results synonymously [32]. Telephone support typically comprises patient follow up, education and counselling delivered via a telephone call made by a specialist nurse. However, patients receiving this form of intervention usually have only mild to moderate CHF symptoms (NYHA class I-II). Remote patient monitoring involves home care of patients using specialist telecare devices to send vital signs directly to the clinician and is often done for patients with severe symptoms of heart failure (NYHA class III-IV) [33].

In reviews that differentiate these approaches and determine the effectiveness of each separately, a technology based approach to patient home monitoring (telemonitoring) is shown to be more effective [34]. In other systematic reviews, telehealth has been compared to a number of alternative approaches, including patient education, specialist (clinician or cardiologist) follow up, nurse home visiting, and telephone support [35–38]. The general conclusion is that telemonitoring alone is insufficient to reduce readmission rates and improve quality of life, and must be integrated with nurse visits and specialist management and follow up, with redesign of the service to support the intervention.

4.3.1 Mortality

Mortality has been the most reported clinical outcome in the study of impact of telehealth to manage CHF. In [39] ten studies reported mortality as a primary outcome, with five studies reporting outcomes with significant significance. However, although the pooled estimate results showed an overall reduction in all-cause mortality, this was not statistically significant (0.77, 0.61 to 0.98, $P = 0.02$). Funnel

	Telemonitoring		Control			Risk Ratio
Study or Subgroup	**Events**	**Total**	**Events**	**Total**	**Weight**	**IV, Fixed, 95% CI**
Antonicelli 2008	3	28	5	29	2.9%	0.62 [0.16, 2.36]
Balk 2008	9	101	8	113	6.2%	1.26 [0.50, 3.14]
Cleland 2005	36	168	28	85	29.2%	0.65 [0.43, 0.99]
Dar 2009	17	91	5	91	5.6%	3.40 [1.31, 8.83]
Giordano 2008	21	230	32	230	19.1%	0.66 [0.39, 1.10]
Goldberg 2003	11	138	26	142	11.6%	0.44 [0.22, 0.85]
Soran 2008	11	160	17	155	9.8%	0.63 [0.30, 1.29]
Wakefields 2008	15	52	11	49	11.3%	1.28 [0.66, 2.52]
Weintraub 2005	1	95	4	93	1.1%	0.24 [0.03, 2.15]
Woodend 2008	5	62	4	59	3.2%	1.19 [0.34, 4.22]
Total (95% CI)		**1125**		**1046**	**100.0%**	**0.77 [0.61, 0.97]**
Total events	129		140			

Heterogeneity: $Chi^2 = 18.39$, df = 9 (P = 0.03); $I^2 = 51\%$
Test for overall effect: Z = 2.25 (P = 0.02)

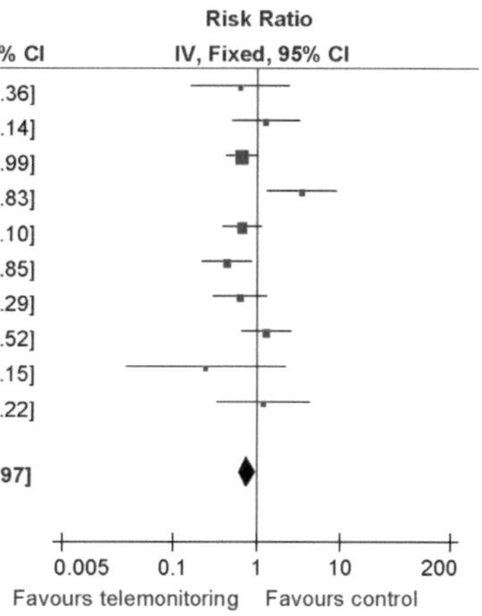

Figure 9.
Effect of telemonitoring on all-cause mortality [39].

plots did not indicate bias, however, heterogeneity was possible (P = 0.03, $I^2 = 51\%$) (**Figure 9**).

4.3.2 Medication adherence

Only 3 studies out of the 11 evaluated the effectiveness of telemonitoring on compliance by patients with their treatment and adherence to medication. The study in [40] reported no significant difference, whereas [41] reported improved compliance with treatment in the telemonitoring group.

4.3.3 Quality of life

The eight studies evaluating quality of life of patients reported no statistically significant general improvement for patients from the intervention. However some studies did report certain aspects of awareness were improved. For example, [42], using SF-36 and MLHF, reported that knowledge about CHF was significantly higher among patients in the intervention group (P < .001). The study in [43] reported significant difference on the vitality subscale of SF-36 at 1 month (P = 0.022), 3 months (P = 0.017) and a year (P = 0.009). Similarly, [44] noted that improvement was achieved over time by using MLHF. [41] reported significant difference in health perception score of SF-36 (P = 0.046). Only two studies assessed anxiety and depression scores. The Minnesota Living with Heart Failure (MLHF) and Short Form (SF-36) Questionnaire were used in all studies to measure Quality of Life.

4.3.4 Managing blood pressure

Blood pressure must be carefully managed in patients with CHF. **Figure 10** shows how telehealth was used to manage reduction of the blood pressure in a patient to an appropriate level [45]. However the blood pressure and pulse rate became erratic. Further investigation determined the patient had atrial fibrillation. Recent blood pressure devices now provide an indication if they determine erratic pulse rate.

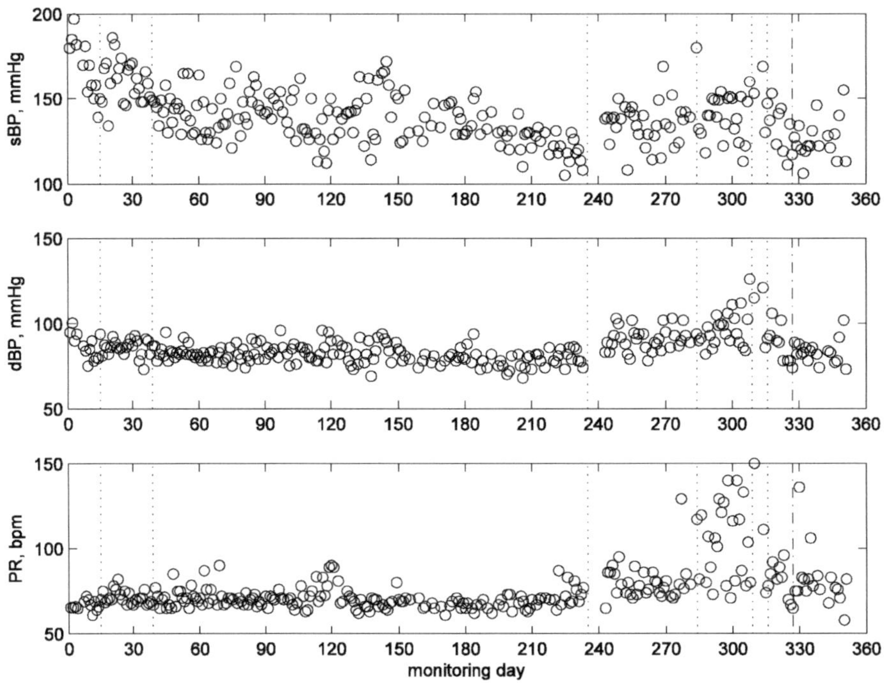

Figure 10.
Daily blood pressure and pulse rate [45].

4.3.5 Monitoring weight

Weight is often monitored in patients with CHF. During exacerbation patients will develop oedema with a corresponding gain in weight. The gain in weight is relatively rapid, over the period of a few days, and the change may be easily detected to generate an alert.

4.4 Clinical benefits in patients with COPD

Chronic obstructive pulmonary disease (COPD), which is characterized by a chronic irreversible airflow limitation, is a leading cause of mortality and morbidity globally and results in substantial costs and healthcare utilisation. Several diseases are categorised as COPD, including asthma, lung disease, and pulmonary fibrosis; each has its own characteristics, progression, and approaches to telehealth have differed accordingly.

4.4.1 Physical activity

Early telehealth approaches concentrated on rehabilitation and used education and intervention via telephone and messaging to encourage patients to perform exercises to improve pulmonary function and increase tolerance to physical activity. Meta-analysis of studies using intervention [46] showed positive outcome for telehealth to increase the duration of physical activity (**Figure 11**), tolerance to 6 minute walk (**Figure 12**), and reduce episodes of dyspnoea (**Figure 13**).

4.4.2 Progression of disease

While effective, such approaches could be considered labour-intensive, especially when continuing to contact patients who are responding. Recent efforts in

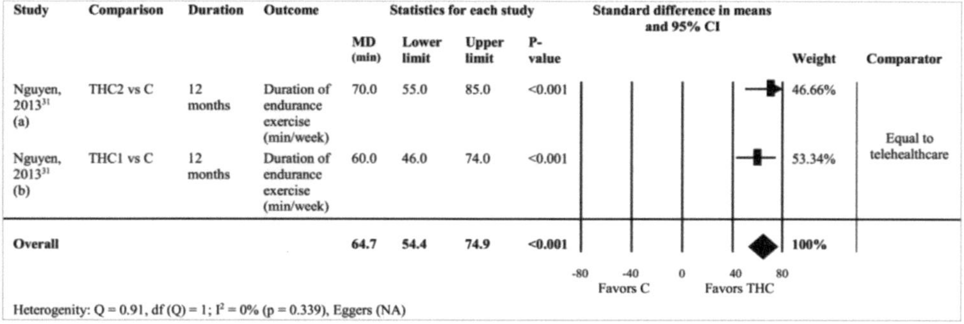

Figure 11.
Forest plot of the effect of telehealth on duration of physical activity [46].

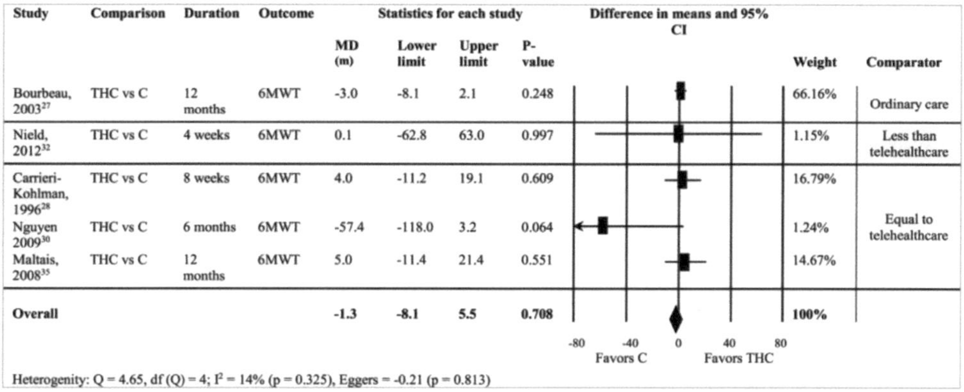

Figure 12.
Forest plot of the effect of telehealth on 6 minute walk [46].

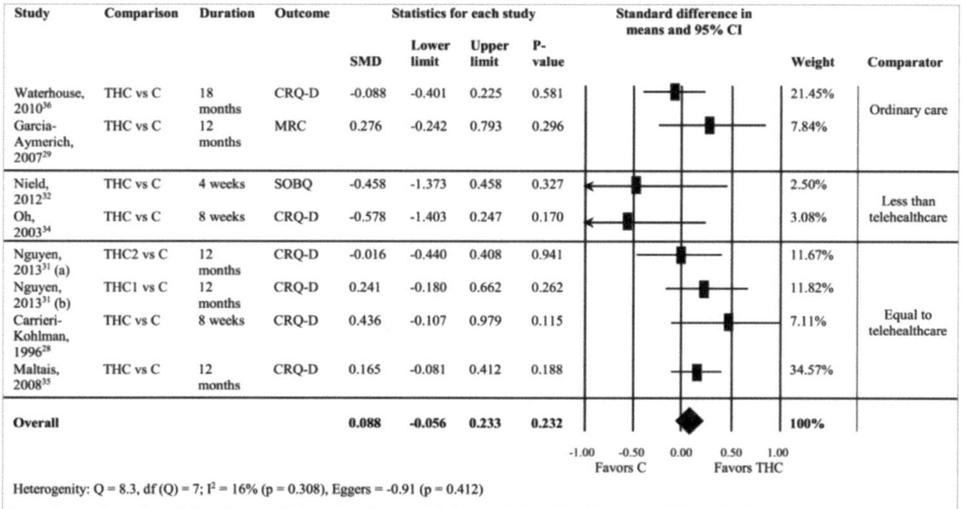

Figure 13.
Forest plot of the effect of telehealth on dyspnoea [46].

telehealth have concentrated on monitoring vital signs to predict exacerbation, primarily measuring daily SpO_2, and concentrate efforts on those in greatest need.

A meta-analysis of studies using vital signs to manage patients with severe COPD [47] shows that there is little change to FEV1; a primary measure of the severity of COPD. As telehealth is not a treatment, and COPD is progressive, then this might be expected. However, every exacerbation can reduce lung function, thus the earlier treatment for the exacerbation is started - the less might be the impact on lung function.

4.4.3 Hospital admission

The same meta-analysis [47] shows that use of telehealth to monitor for exacerbation in COPD can reduce the number of emergency room (ER) visits (**Figure 14**), however the number of hospitalisations was not significantly reduced (**Figure 15**)

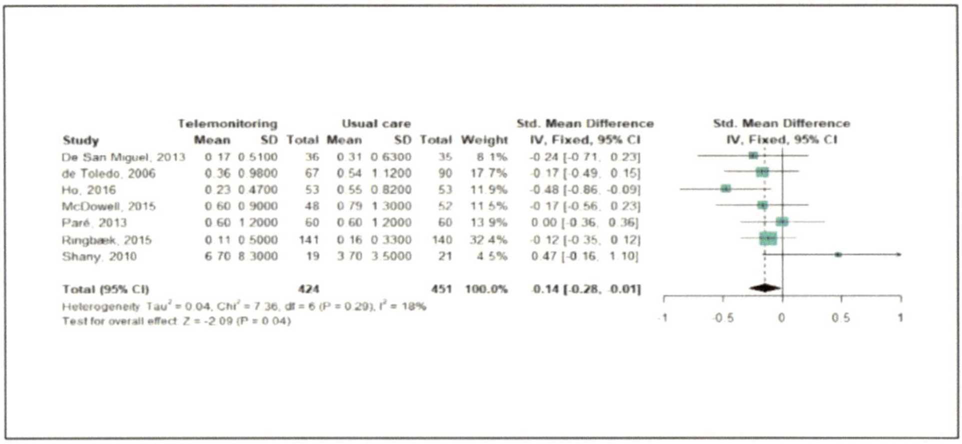

Figure 14.
Forest plot for the effectiveness of telemonitoring for decreasing the number of ER visits due to severe COPD exacerbations [47].

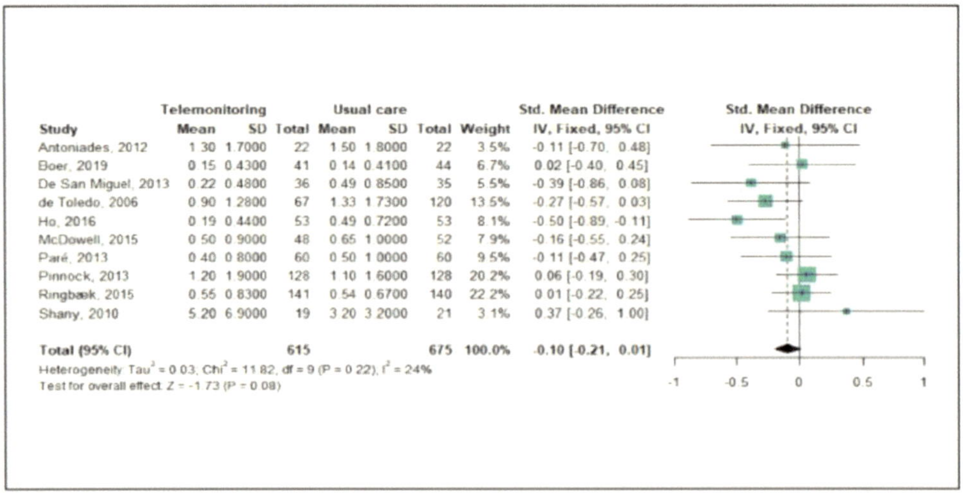

Figure 15.
Forest plot of the effectiveness of telemonitoring for decreasing the number of hospitalisations due to severe COPD exacerbations. [47].

and thus there was no effect on the number of exacerbations. Similar results were reported in a study on cost-effectiveness [48], however the length of stay was reduced and thus there may be benefit from the earlier intervention permitted by telehealth.

4.4.4 Monitoring pulse oximetry

Blood oxygen (SpO_2) is the most often monitored parameter in patients with COPD. In general, COPD patients have a blood oxygen level that is lower than normal, but is maintained and the patient becomes accustomed. During exacerbation the level will fall, and a threshold may be set to generate an alert. **Figure 16** [45] shows SpO_2 measurements for a typical COPD patient, the vertical dotted lines indicate clinical events. SpO_2 is seen to fall at these times. However SpO_2 also falls at other times, which would generate false alerts. Improved algorithms are required to improve accuracy.

4.5 Clinical benefits in patients with diabetes

Diabetes is a disease in which a patient is unable to produce sufficient insulin to control the level of glucose in their blood. In Type I and insulin-dependent Type II, patients produce little or no insulin, and so must inject insulin to meet their need to maintain their blood glucose level with limits. The amount of insulin to be injected to maintain the level of blood glucose is determined by the patient by taking a measurement of their current blood glucose and calculating the amount of carbohydrate they about to ingest.

Type II patients may be able to manage their level of blood glucose by diet and exercise alone, or require an increasing level of oral therapy as their condition deteriorates until they will be required to inject insulin.

Telehealth has been applied to the management of patients with diabetes in many projects, including Type I, Type II and both forms. In addition, many approaches to telehealth have been used to facilitate early detection and diagnosis, monitor disease progression, and provide management. Methods include telemonitoring, teleconsultation, interventions delivered by computer, and combinations.

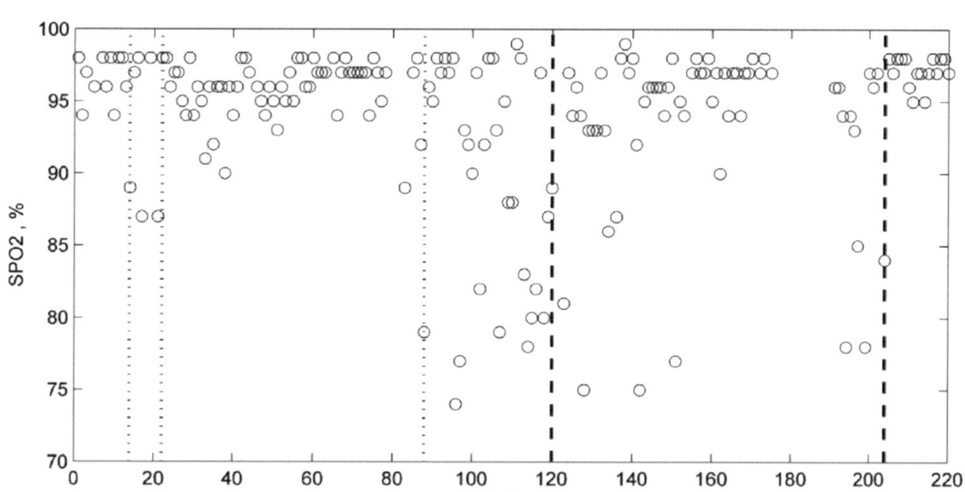

Figure 16.
Pulse oximetry in COPD patients [45].

4.5.1 Type II diabetes

The primary outcome of studies is the level of Hb1Ac, which provides a measure of the long-term level of blood glucose. It is the primary means of routine management of patients with diabetes, with the aim to bring within a target range. Daily fasting glucose may also be measured as an outcome, with the aim to maintain within a target range. A secondary outcome is blood pressure, as it is important that this is well maintained in order to prevent complications of the disease, and this may be controlled in studies. Further secondary outcomes include lipid levels, which would include cholesterol and low density lipoprotein and high density lipoprotein also to prevent complications of the disease, and may also be controlled in a study.

One meta-analysis [49] analyses the outcome from each approach separately. The analysis (**Figure 17**) shows that each approach, other than telecase-management and telemonitoring that were marginal, achieved similar outcome that was a positive outcome for telehealth, although telecase-management with teleconsultation achieved a higher average outcome but with large variation. In part, this outcome can be explained because patients have the goal to reach a target within a specified range and once attained no further change is expected or required. This will limit the mean difference, which will also be influenced by the baseline.

The meta-analysis [49] also analyses each of the secondary outcomes by approach. Secondary outcomes were generally similar between telehealth and standard care; however this will be dependent on the protocol for intervention.

Other systematic reviews and meta-analysis agree with these outcomes: [50] reports a mean reduction of 0.17% in HbA1c in telehealth compared to usual care, especially for patients with mean baseline greater than 8.0%. However, there was no clinically significant reduction in LDL-cholesterol (LDL-c), body mass index (BMI), systolic (SBP) or diastolic blood pressure (DBP); [51] reports mean reduction between 0.2% and 0.64%, with a pooled mean of 0.39% in HbA1c; [52] reports mean reduction of 0.486% in HbA1c and some improvements in secondary outcomes such as diastolic blood pressure and body mass index (**Figure 18**).

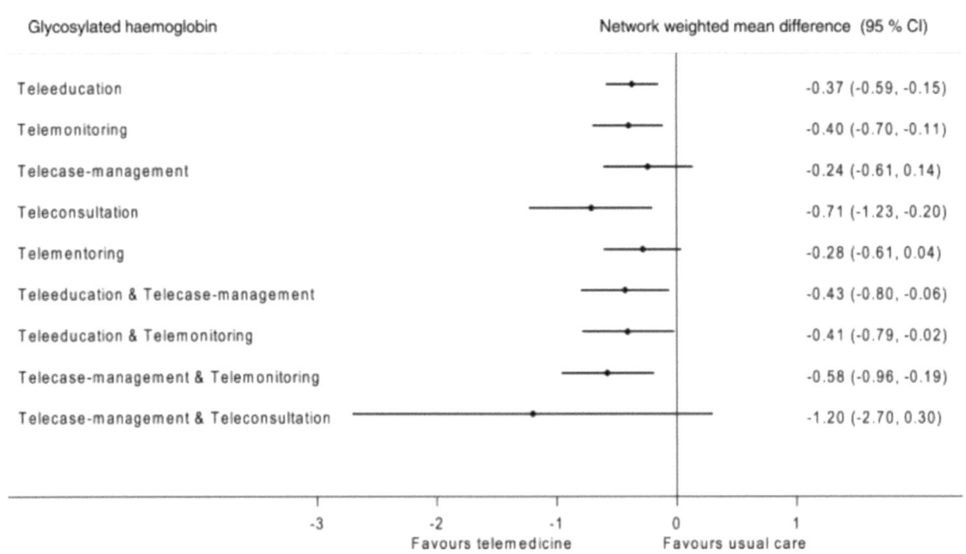

Figure 17.
Change in glycated haemoglobin in adults with Type II diabetes by telehealth approach [49].

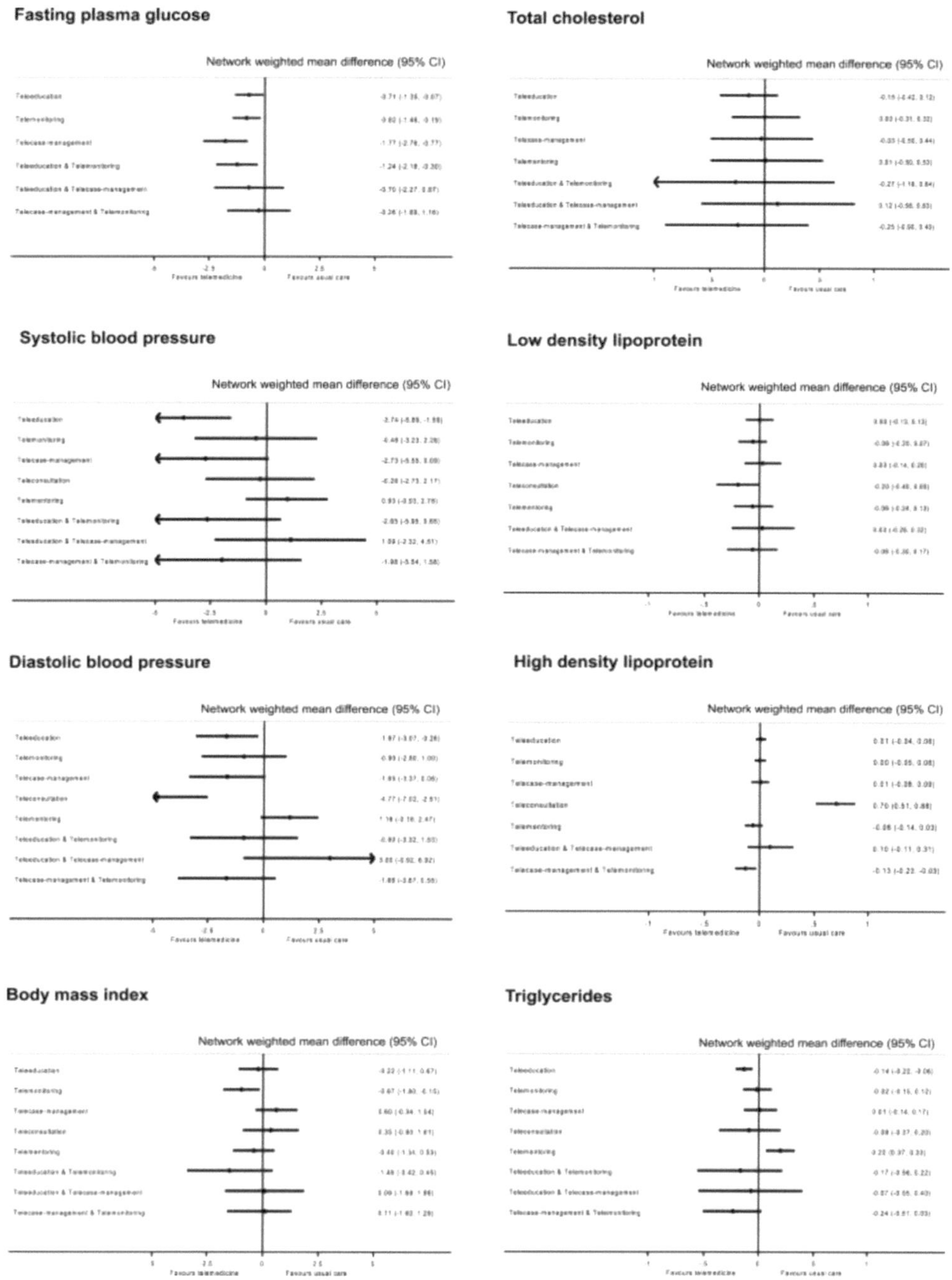

Figure 18.
Change in secondary cardiovascular outcomes of different telehealth strategies compared to usual care in adults with Type II diabetes by telehealth approach [49].

4.5.2 Intervention strategies

Most studies on telehealth are conducted on a selected group of patients that is considered homogeneous and outcomes are considered through statistical measures. One study investigated management of all patients with diabetes in a primary care setting [53], performing two weeks of monitoring daily blood glucose and blood pressure, repeated every 6 months following the UK national framework. Data from each patient was reviewed to assess whether their condition was well controlled, and if not, intervention was used to manage the condition and establish correct control. The study identified three distinct patient groups: the well-controlled who required no intervention; patients requiring intervention to re-establish control; and patients in denial.

The well-controlled patients were aware of their condition, and managed their lifestyle and medication accordingly. They required no intervention. The daily measurements provided by the telemonitoring gave insight into the habits of the patients who required intervention and allowed directed and personalised intervention strategies, for example by identifying patients who did not follow diet at the weekend as part of a social activity, seen as a spike in daily glucose. The daily measurements also clearly identified patients who were in denial, frequently not taking any medication, and the data could be used to confront the patient in order to encourage change. Monitoring would continue until correct management was established. 37% of the patients were identified as needing intervention, resulting in a mean reduction in HbA1c of 3 mmol/mol and mean reduction in systolic blood pressure of 5 mmHg.

The short period of intervention was considered more effective than continuous monitoring of patients who were well managed. It was expected that patients would comply initially but then lapse after a period, when the monitoring would be repeated.

4.5.3 Type I diabetes

In Type I and insulin dependent Type II diabetes the goals for control of blood glucose are somewhat different. In addition to achieving a long term average, as indicated by HbA1c, within the target range, a patient with Type I diabetes must maintain their blood glucose within a target range at all times through injection of an appropriate amount of insulin to match their current blood glucose level, activity and ingestion of food. This requires frequent measurement of their blood glucose. Traditionally this has been through regular use of a finger prick and a glucose meter, usually measured before a meal to determine the required amount of insulin. Post-prandial measurements may be taken to monitor correct management. Glucose meters typically store many measurements that may be uploaded to a monitoring service for review by the clinician and telehealth service.

One meta-analysis study [54] compares separately the outcome from studies that included Type I and Type II patients. The outcomes show improvement in mean change to HbA1c in each of the three categories that were studied, Type I and Type II, Type I, and Type II (**Figure 19**); the Type II group achieving the greatest change.

4.5.4 Continuous glucose monitoring

A recent development in telehealth is the introduction of devices that can be placed on the body to monitor blood glucose on a continuous basis. Improvements in biomaterials have extended the time that the sensor remains on the body to 10 days [55]. These devices can communicate their data to a monitoring application that may be used by the patient directly to monitor their blood glucose to determine insulin dose, and detect and provide an alert when the blood glucose level goes outside thresholds. Data may also be forwarded to others monitoring the patient that includes the parents of juvenile diabetes patients and the clinician.

Studies [56, 57] have shown that continuous glucose monitoring (CGM) can reduce HbA1c in Type II patients (**Figure 20**); although it is not clear if CGM produces improved reduction in HbA1c compared to other telehealth approaches.

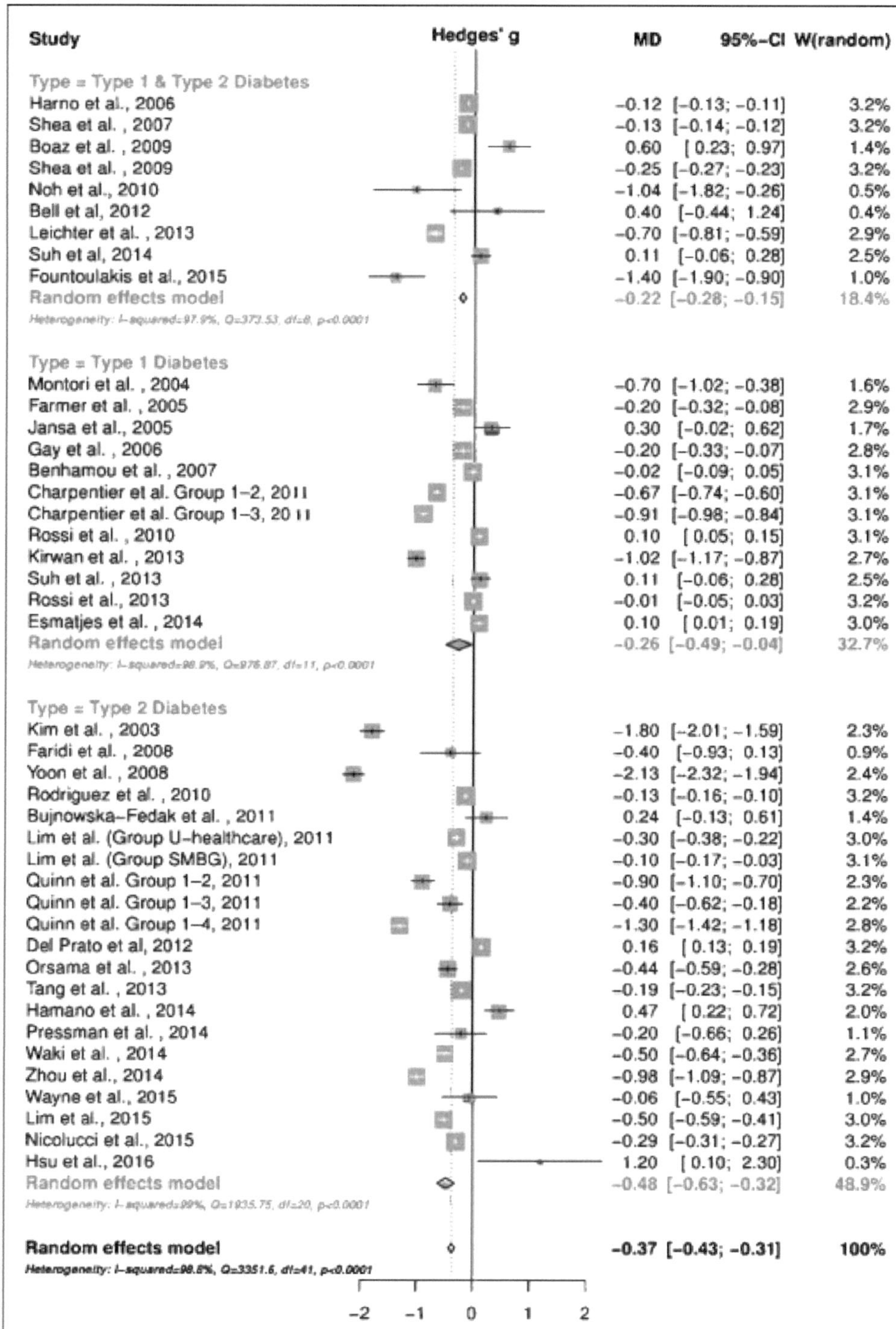

Figure 19.
Mean difference in the changes in HbA1c levels for telehealth and usual care [54].

The most valuable use of CGM is in the management of Type I and insulin dependent Type II patients as it improves short-term control, provides alerts of high and low values (hyperglycaemia and hypoglycaemia). This reduces the number of times a finger prick is required, reducing scarring and the incorrect results from taking blood from over-used sites.

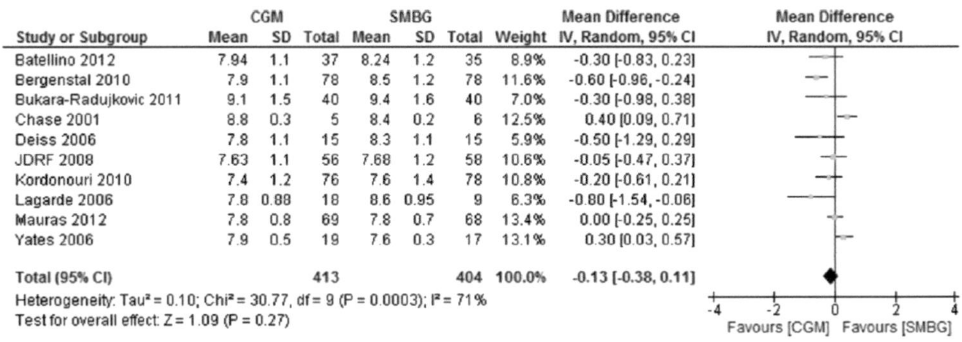

Figure 20.
Mean difference in the changes in HbA1c levels for telehealth using CGM [56].

4.6 Clinical benefits in patients with hypertension

Hypertension is a disease in which a patient has an elevated level of blood pressure. It is normally managed using drug therapy. Telehealth has often been proposed as a method to manage patients with hypertension.

A meta-analysis [58] of the use of telehealth versus usual office management of hypertension shows a statistically significant reduction of both systolic (3.4 mmHg) (**Figure 21**) and diastolic (1.6 mmHg) (**Figure 22**) blood pressure in patients managed by telehealth, however the reduction is not of clinical significance.

Again this outcome may be explained by the target being to bring patients within a threshold. Given the range of patients between those well-managed, in need of intervention, and in denial, overall outcome may be small, but impact on a small number of patients may significant. Telehealth allows resource to be targeted to those in most need.

Telehealth in management of hypertension probably has greatest effect when used with the newly diagnosed, and allows rapid titration of medication to bring them below threshold, without need for frequent visits to the clinician, especially

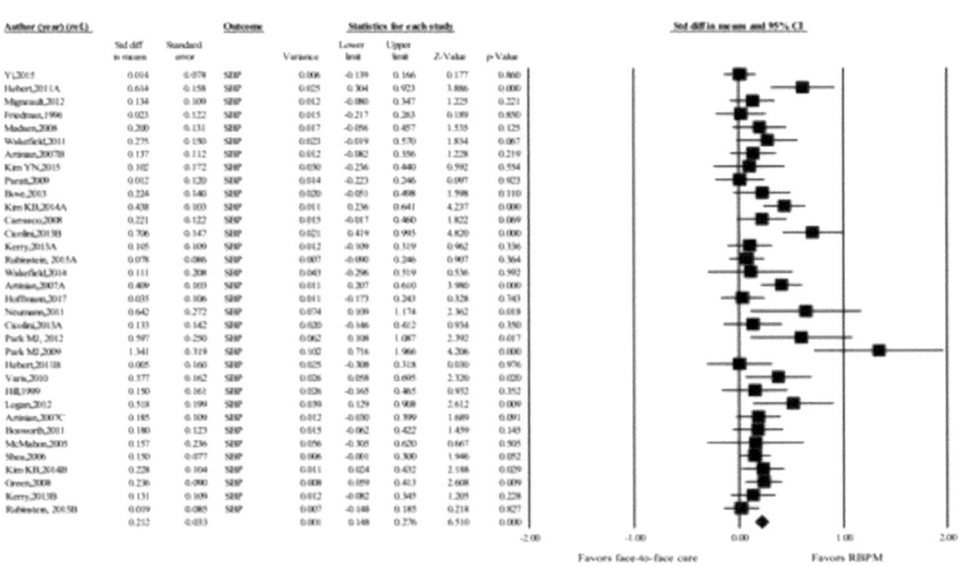

Figure 21.
Mean difference in the changes in Systolic Blood Pressure [58].

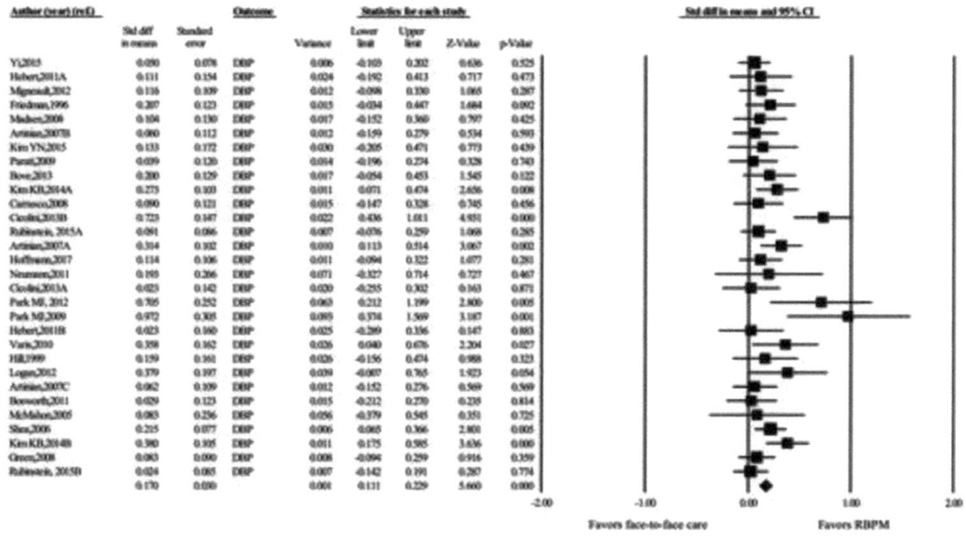

Figure 22.
Mean difference in the changes in Diastolic Blood Pressure [58].

valuable where the patient must travel a large distance. Once the patient becomes well-managed, the need for telehealth is significantly reduced and could be removed.

Telehealth has also found a place in diagnosing hypertension. The elevated blood pressure measured in the clinician office is a well-known phenomenon and can mask the presence of hypertension. Ambulatory blood pressure has been used in the past to confirm the diagnosis. Telehealth, monitoring daily blood pressure at home for a short period, has become accepted as an alternative method for diagnosis.

4.7 Clinical benefits in pregnancy

Several conditions can develop during pregnancy, including gestational diabetes and pre-eclampsia. In general, these conditions resolve postpartum, however it is important that they are monitored carefully until fully resolved. Usual care is frequent monitoring at the out-patient clinic of the maternity hospital, requiring travel with a new-born baby, and possibly other young children. Telehealth offers the means to undertake the monitoring at home.

4.7.1 Gestational diabetes

Gestational diabetes is a short term condition which may develop during pregnancy and will generally resolve postpartum. Good control of blood glucose is essential for correct development of the foetus, as high blood glucose severely impacts birth weight. Monitoring and management strategy is the same as Type II diabetes.

Conclusions from meta-analysis of the outcomes of studies of telehealth to manage gestational diabetes are mixed. One study [59] concludes glycaemic control (HbA1c, pre and postprandial blood glucose) to be similar between the telehealth and usual care groups, although face-to-face and unscheduled consultations were reduced. However, another study [60] determined significant improvement in glycaemic control in HbA1c (**Figure 23A**), pre-prandial blood glucose (**Figure 23B**) and 2 hour postprandial blood glucose (**Figure 23C**).

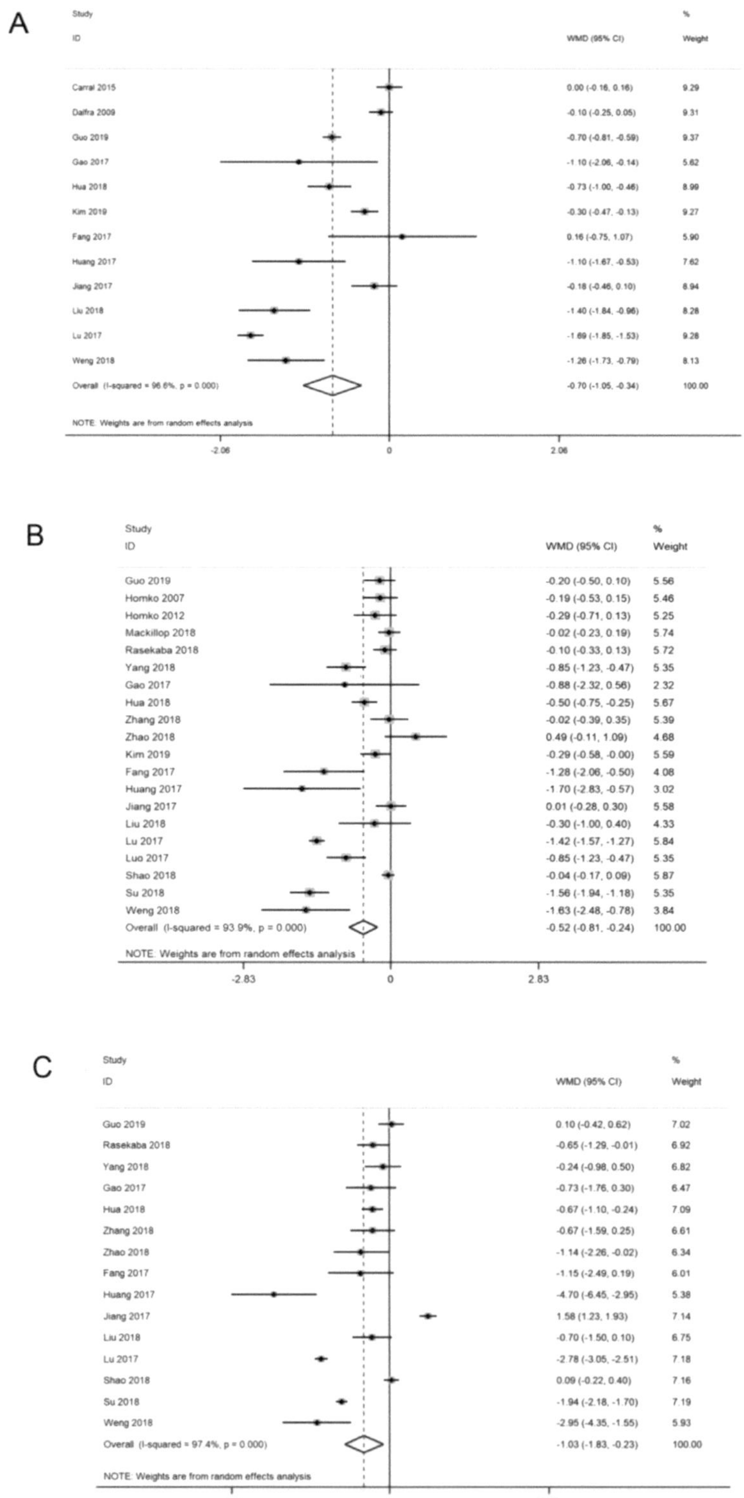

Figure 23.
Mean difference in the changes in (A) HbA1c, (B) FBG (C) 2hBG [60].

4.7.2 Pre-eclampsia

Pre-eclampsia is a serious condition that usually develops late in pregnancy and will necessitate early delivery. It is associated with high blood pressure. The condition normally resolves quickly postpartum, and management is to check the blood pressure periodically until it returns to normal value. Telehealth has been used to monitor blood pressure in pre-eclampsia. Blood pressure may also be monitored during pregnancy in those at high risk of developing pre-eclampsia [61].

There are fewer reported outcomes for studies in pre-eclampsia than other uses of telehealth. The one systematic review [62] reports that telehealth is liked by participants, but there is little difference in mean blood pressure between telehealth and usual care. This is to be expected as telehealth is being used to replace visits to the clinic and provide convenience for the patient.

4.8 Clinical benefits in patients with other diseases

Use of telehealth has been reported for the management of other diseases, such as monitoring patients during the acute phase of a disease (sometimes called hospital at home), recovery and release from hospital, rehabilitation, and in high acuity settings such as specialist residential homes. For example, in [63] ECG recordings taken from residents feeling unwell in residential homes were used to recognise cardiac tamponade in one instance and myocardial infarction in a second, which allowed prompt intervention and management.

4.9 Health and wellness

Health and wellness is an often considered area for telehealth. This would be typified by the wearing of a "smart" watch that includes capability to perform measurements of pulse oximetry at the wrist, which may be used to determine the level of blood oxygen and heart rate. Devices may also include sensors to count steps, GPS to determine distance covered, and timers to monitor periods of exercise. Whilst such monitoring may be of interest to the individual and may influence adoption of improved lifestyle and impact on health, there is little evidence that this type of monitoring provides data with clinical value, as often the data is unreliable and of poor quality.

There are efforts to integrate similar sensors within clothing, but there are practical problems in where the sensors can be placed conveniently and provide meaningful and reliable clinical measurements.

Most frequently sensors are integrated in a chest belt of some form, which can then monitor ECG and respiration. This has been implemented as a vest, but most patients do not like the constricted feel. For women, it can be integrated into items such as the bra.

5. Service benefits

5.1 Service redesign

For telehealth to be most effective, great care must be given to the way in which the service is established; this includes consideration of the patient care pathway, workflow, information flow and professional relationships. For cost-effective reasons, management and care of patients is often transferred to services in the community and primary care.

Therefore the design of the telehealth service must include assigning responsibilities for regular checking of data, making decisions on management and therapy, referral, and release from hospital. There must also be education and training for staff in community and primary care to prepare them for new responsibilities and managing complex conditions. The telehealth service must be provided with strong management that establishes good relationships between all clinicians, and has clear plans for change management.

Business Process Modelling (BPM) can be an effective methodology to capture patient care pathway, workflow and information flow, in order to understand the existing service model, and to provide understanding of the optimum structure to integrate telehealth.

Figure 24 [64] demonstrates how the components and information flows of a telehealth system may be captured and elements of the workflow depicted. This model may then be used to determine how the services are established to enact the requirements identified by the model.

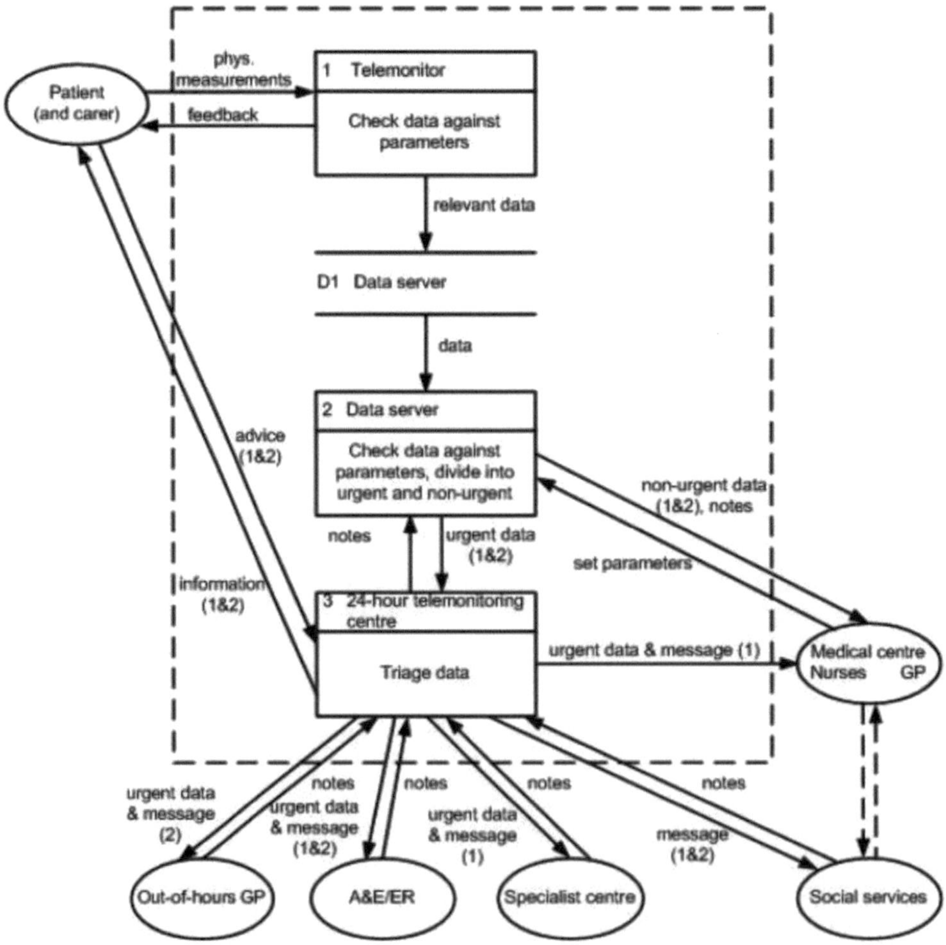

Figure 24.
Optimum design of a telehealth system in the UK (1) During office hours; (2) Out of hours [64].

5.2 Cost benefit analysis

Cost benefit analysis in health is complex as it has to consider not only financial aspects (incremental cost), but also the benefits in quality life that society would expect to be given to the patient (incremental benefit). **Figure 25** shows how the analysis of economic aspects is based on the two axes of increased cost and increased benefit. This gives rise to the four quadrants with their respective consideration for a decision. Decisions in the upper left quadrant and lower right quadrant are straight-forward as they can be made on a financial basis. Decisions in the other two quadrants must include a consideration of a combination of financial and patient benefit. As these carry a societal aspect that may be difficult to quantify, patient benefit is assessed in financial terms in health economics.

The approach adopted is to determine the impact to the quality of life of the patient (e.g. hip replacement gives mobility) and how it is maintained over time. This methodology is termed the Quality Adjusted Life Year, and the aggregate of the benefit over the baseline over time is determined (**Figure 26**). A notional cost is assigned to achieve a QALY (e.g. £30,000 per QALY). This allows the cost–benefit analysis to be made on an economic basis and a decision made.

However, studies do not show telehealth provides significant impact on quality of life, thus there is little change in incremental benefit and analysis concentrates on incremental cost, or cost-effectiveness.

5.3 Cost-effectiveness

Analysis of cost-effectiveness of telehealth requires study of the impact on use of all the health services by patients. This normally focusses on hospital services, such

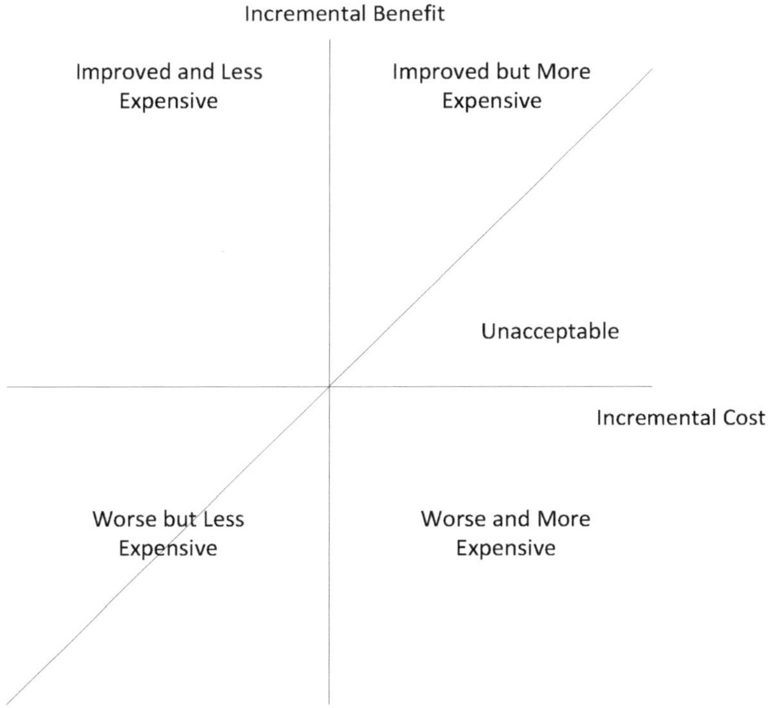

Figure 25.
Cost–benefit analysis.

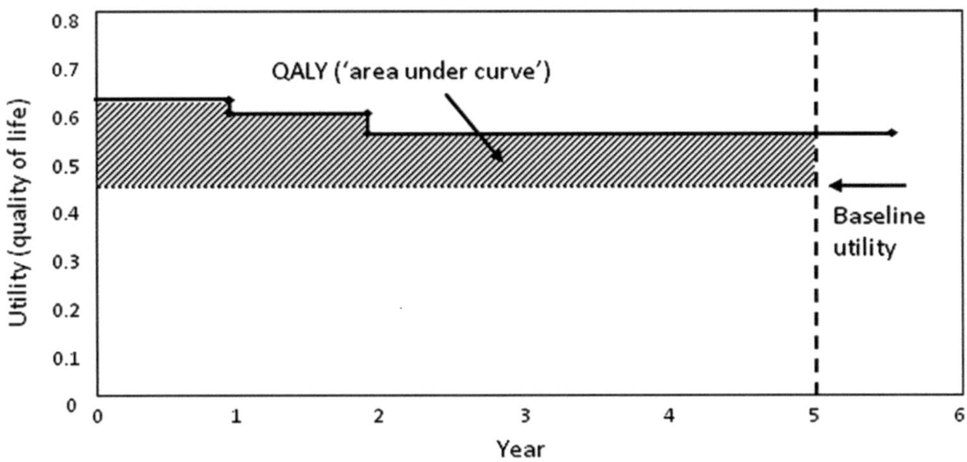

Figure 26.
Use of the QALY to assess cost benefit.

as admission, emergency room visits, and length of stay, as these contribute most. This is balanced by the incremental cost of the technology and staffing costs to provide the service. A cost model may then be created to evaluate. However few well defined studies exist. The review in [39] provides a meta-analysis of the impact on hospital services for patients with CHF; however none of the studies provided outcomes for cost-effectiveness.

5.3.1 All cause and CHF hospital admission

The same review [39] found six studies that reported all cause hospital admissions as primary outcome (**Figure 27**). None reported significant reduction and the pooled estimates support this (0.99, 0.88 to 1.11, P = 0.84).

In contrast, some reduction in CHF hospital admission was reported by the same set of studies (**Figure 28**). Pooled estimates of the given data indicate that there is a small reduction that is significantly relevant (0.73, 0.62 to 0.87, P = 0.0004). Bias was unlikely but possibility of heterogeneity could not be ruled out in all cause hospital admission (P = 0.03, I^2 = 59%). There was little evidence of heterogeneity for CHF (P = 0.44, I^2 = 0%).

	Telemonitoring		Control			Risk Ratio
Study or Subgroup	Events	Total	Events	Total	Weight	IV, Fixed, 95% CI
Cleland 2005	75	168	40	85	16.1%	0.95 [0.72, 1.26]
Dar 2009	33	91	23	91	6.4%	1.43 [0.92, 2.24]
Giordano 2008	67	230	96	230	19.9%	0.70 [0.54, 0.90]
Goldberg 2003	65	138	67	142	20.7%	1.00 [0.78, 1.28]
Mortara 2009	106	301	48	160	16.0%	1.17 [0.89, 1.56]
Soran 2008	75	160	66	155	21.0%	1.10 [0.86, 1.41]
Total (95% CI)		1088		863	100.0%	0.99 [0.88, 1.11]
Total events	421		340			

Heterogeneity: Chi² = 12.21, df = 5 (P = 0.03); I² = 59%
Test for overall effect: Z = 0.20 (P = 0.84)

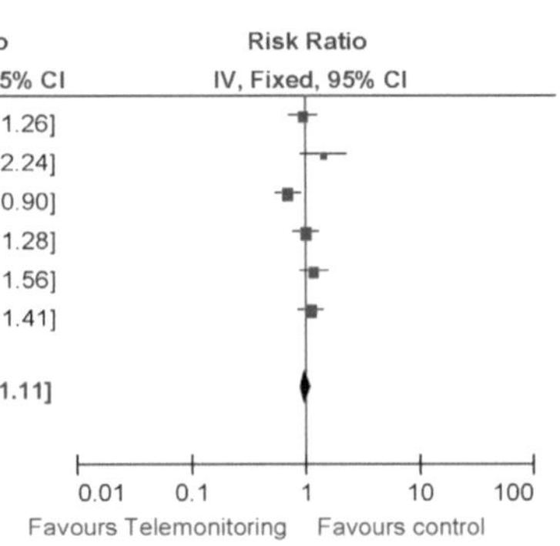

Figure 27.
Effect of telemonitoring on all-cause hospital admission [39].

Study or Subgroup	Telemonitorig Events	Telemonitorig Total	Control Events	Control Total	Weight	Risk Ratio IV, Fixed, 95% CI
Cleland 2005	38	168	23	85	14.9%	0.84 [0.53, 1.31]
Dar 2009	10	91	17	91	5.7%	0.59 [0.28, 1.21]
Giordano 2008	43	230	73	230	27.5%	0.59 [0.42, 0.82]
Mortara 2009	53	301	28	160	17.3%	1.01 [0.66, 1.52]
Soran 2008	30	160	37	155	16.3%	0.79 [0.51, 1.20]
Wakefields 2008	21	52	29	49	18.3%	0.68 [0.46, 1.02]
Total (95% CI)		**1002**		**770**	**100.0%**	**0.73 [0.62, 0.87]**
Total events	195		207			

Heterogeneity: Chi² = 4.83, df = 5 (P = 0.44); I² = 0%
Test for overall effect: Z = 3.52 (P = 0.0004)

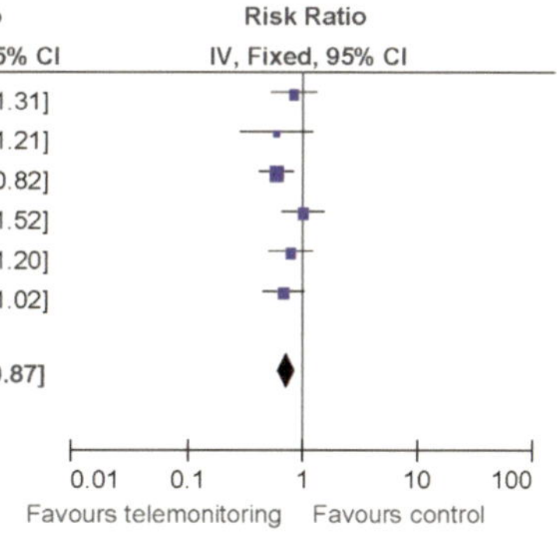

Figure 28.
Effect of telemonitoring on CHF hospital admission [39].

5.3.2 Emergency room visits

The review [39] found seven studies that provided the number of emergency visits as secondary outcome (**Figure 29**); but with mixed outcome. Some studies observed no significant difference in emergency visits among the patients in treatment and control arm (P = 0.43); some reported lower emergency contacts were observed; yet others reported an increase in emergency room visits. Pooled results of data extracted from 4 studies showed no significant reduction in risk of emergency admission between the groups (1.04, 0.86 to 1.26). Heterogeneity exited as P = 0.001, I^2 = 82%.

5.3.3 Length of stay

The review [39] found nine studies that evaluated the effect of intervention on length of stay in hospital. Among these, seven studies showed no difference in length of stay at hospital due to any cause or CHF among the patients across both groups. Two studies reported reduction in length of stay among patients in home monitoring group due to CHF.

However a more detailed analysis on length of stay [48] reveals that patients with CHF who are admitted to hospital often present a complex set of issues. Patients sometimes develop complications and so remain in hospital for an extended period; likewise, earlier admissions may have been protracted, but stays during the trial are significantly shortened; this results in a significant spread in length of stay (**Figure 30**). Overall a reduction in length of stay is observed. This is often attributed to early discharge being possible as the patient feels safe to return

Study or Subgroup	Telemonitoring Events	Telemonitoring Total	Control Events	Control Total	Weight	Risk Ratio IV, Fixed, 95% CI
Cleland 2005	67	168	13	85	12.2%	2.61 [1.53, 4.45]
Dansky 2008	14	45	40	112	13.9%	0.87 [0.53, 1.44]
Dar 2009	20	91	32	91	15.3%	0.63 [0.39, 1.01]
Soran 2008	73	160	69	155	58.6%	1.02 [0.80, 1.31]
Total (95% CI)		**464**		**443**	**100.0%**	**1.04 [0.86, 1.26]**
Total events	174		154			

Heterogeneity: Chi² = 16.27, df = 3 (P = 0.0010); I² = 82%
Test for overall effect: Z = 0.43 (P = 0.67)

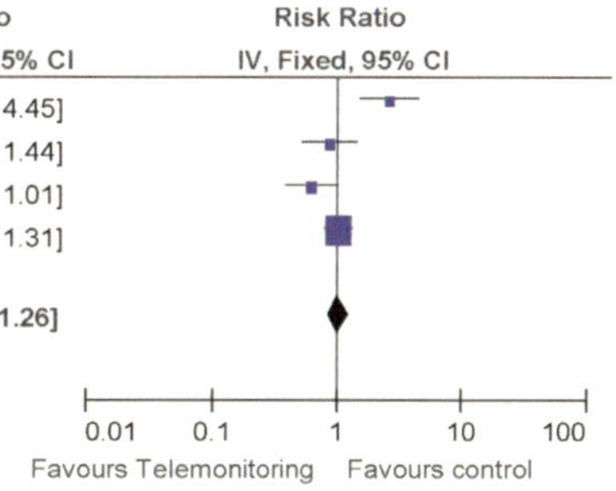

Figure 29.
Effect of telemonitoring on all-cause emergency room visit [39].

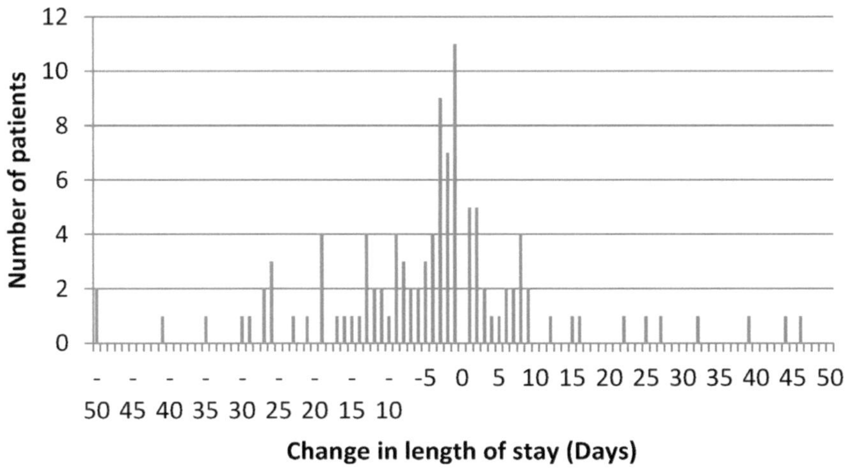

Figure 30.
Change in length of stay for each patient compared to length of stay in the period immediately before monitoring [48].

home because they are being monitored. There may be an affect due to the earlier planned admission and the prompt intervention results in reduced recovery time.

5.3.4 Cost

Two of the studies in the meta-analysis [39] evaluated the cost effectiveness of a telemonitoring based intervention against the usual care but neither determined that there was a reduction. One study on cost-effectiveness [48] undertook evaluation on two separate organisations (Primary Care Trusts) and found wide discrepancy in outcomes, indicating why the literature is inconclusive. The study determined an average annual saving of £1023 per patient, but this was highly influenced by factors pertaining to the way in which the service was established and patients were managed.

6. Future developments

6.1 Monitoring activities of daily living

An area of development for telehealth is in monitoring the activities of daily living (ADL), especially of the frail elderly. Changes in behaviour may be used to detect early deterioration in health and before it may be evident in other symptoms, which may also be being monitored by telehealth. This remains a little researched area, with almost all reported work being on development of sensors [65]. However, one of the few studies that reports ADL and correlates with clinical events [45] presents evidence that shows that deviation from an established, characteristic behaviour pattern can indicate deterioration in a health condition and impending clinical event. Anecdotal evidence suggests patients may tire easily and thus rest more in a chair; have altered sleeping patterns; become restless at night; sleep in the day; visit the toilet more frequently; and take longer to complete everyday activities. Simple sensors such as motion and bed/chair occupancy and analysis of their data can be used to monitor these events, patterns of normal behaviour can be established, and deviation can be recognised.

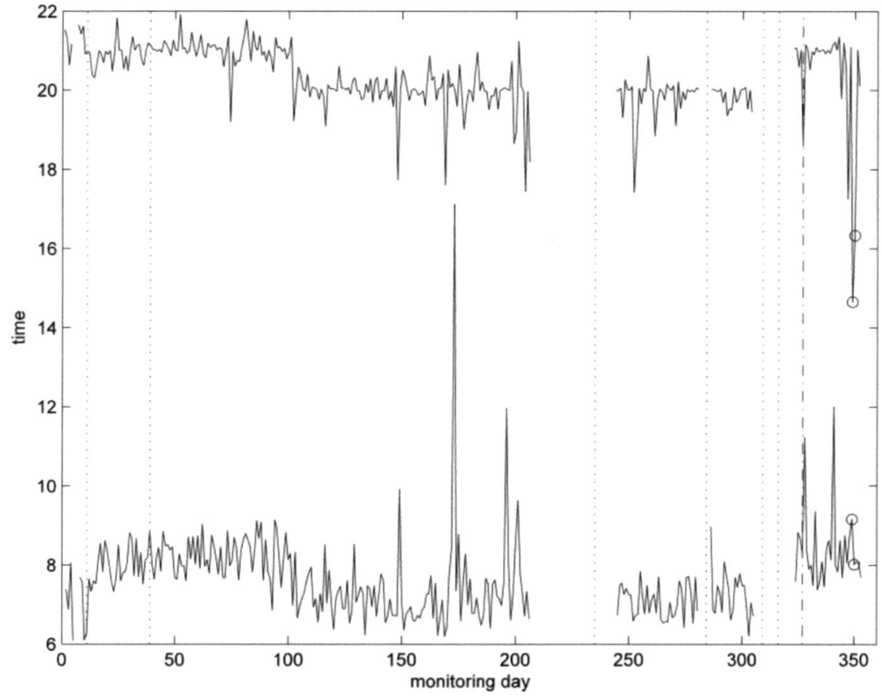

Figure 31.
Time of first and last detected motion in living room [45].

In one example (**Figure 31**), the time of first and last motion in the living room is determined, from which the regular bed and waking time can be inferred. On some days, there is a much later time of waking and earlier bed-time. Naturally caution is required in interpretation of such events, as differences may be easily explained by events such as a trip away from home.

Figure 32 shows the bed occupancy of a patient with pulmonary fibrosis. The black bar shows the time in bed each day. In this example, the patient continued to go to bed around 23:00 each day, but during times of deterioration the patient started to wake earlier, and as severity of the conditioned worsened they had less sleep.

A similar pattern of disturbed sleep was observed in COPD patients during periods of low blood oxygen as indicated in **Figure 33**.

6.2 Technology developments

Technology for telehealth continues to evolve, improve and be developed. This would include sensors becoming lighter, smaller and the emergence of new types of sensor. Technology continues to improve with microcontrollers becoming more powerful, faster, and use less power, at the same time batteries give greater periods of use. This has made possible an explosion in the availability of wearable devices, particular wrist-worn, that can monitor heart rate, blood oxygen and capture ECG.

Chemistry and biomaterials continue to improve, allowing longer periods of use and providing sensors with greater accuracy in applications such as continuous glucose monitoring.

Wireless technology continues to evolve, with improvements to the range and reductions in power. This allows devices based on technologies such as Bluetooth to operate for longer or use smaller batteries. Likewise improvements in mobile

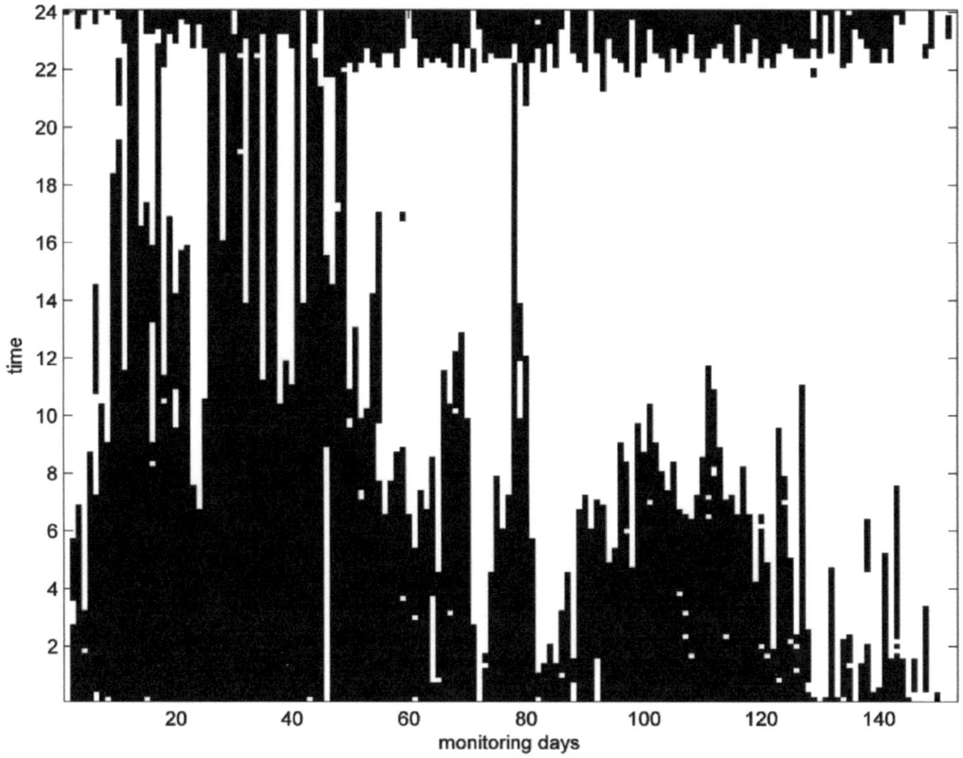

Figure 32.
Daily bed occupancy [45].

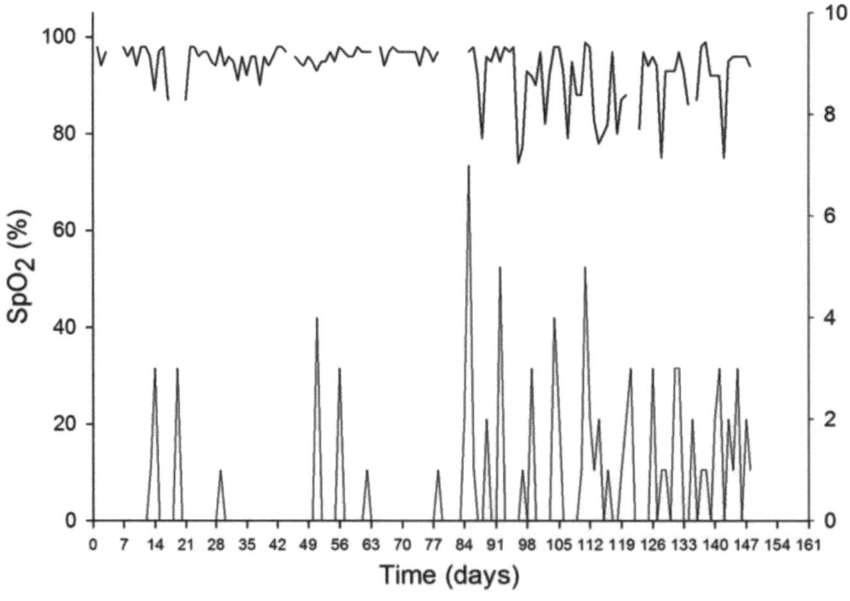

Figure 33.
Incidence of disturbed sleep and low blood oxygen [45].

technology are introducing a range of low-power long range services such as NB-IoT and CAT-M that support direct transmission of data from a device and provide extended battery life.

Telehealth remains beset with devices using proprietary protocols. Although devices may claim to use BlueTooth Low Energy (BLE) as wireless, the data and its format differ significantly between devices and device manufacturers. This locks users into specific devices and applications, which may be acceptable for the consumer market. However it makes it difficult to integrate several devices into a platform to monitor a condition, and many types of device to monitor comorbidities. It also introduces uncertainty to the market regarding continued availability of devices, with consequent loss of investment if a system must be replaced if devices are no longer available.

The situation is not improved by the small number of separate profiles that have been developed for individual medical devices by BlueTooth, and that are fixed in capability. This prevents extensibility and results in proprietary protocols.

There is a great need for protocols that provide semantic interoperability between devices and that are extensible and flexible. The IEEE 11073-20601 [22] base protocol standard and its family of specialisations (IEEE 11073-104xx) with its use of IEEE 11073-10101 nomenclature achieved this goal [66], and is further supported by transparent mapping into enterprise health standards such as IHE PCD-01 and FHIR. However this standard has not been adopted commercially, therefore work has commenced to develop a standard (IEEE 11073-10206) that is based on an abstract version of the object models of IEEE 11073-20601 and that may be used as a guideline to develop other protocols, such as a profile of BLE, that will be semantically interoperable across technologies and thus map transparently to enterprise health standards.

6.3 Algorithms, artificial intelligence and machine learning

Algorithms, artificial intelligence (AI) and machine learning (ML) have been slow to be applied to telehealth. Most telehealth systems continue to use simple thresholds on vital signs data to determine patients at risk of deterioration, which has been shown to have poor performance, resulting in such frequent false alerts that they are often disabled by users and alerts are missed [67].

Patients with COPD often adapt to their condition and will tolerate significantly lower levels of blood oxygen without perceived difference to their health or impact on everyday activities. A simple threshold would determine such patients at risk of deterioration.

Figure 34 shows the daily SpO_2 time-series data for a patient with COPD and the wide variation that is typically observed; short term and long term average are shown, and the vertical dotted lines indicate clinical event.

Using a simple threshold would result in both false negative (value below threshold without clinical event) and false positive (value above threshold during clinical event) indications for this patient.

However when the residual (difference between actual and average) is analysed [68], significant variation is observed, and the standard deviation of the residual is seen to increase significantly during periods of exacerbation (**Figure 35**). Physiologically this might be explained by the patient having a coping mechanism for low blood oxygen, but during exacerbation, this mechanism is overwhelmed or fails, and results in the large variations that are observed, giving a clearer indication of impending deterioration.

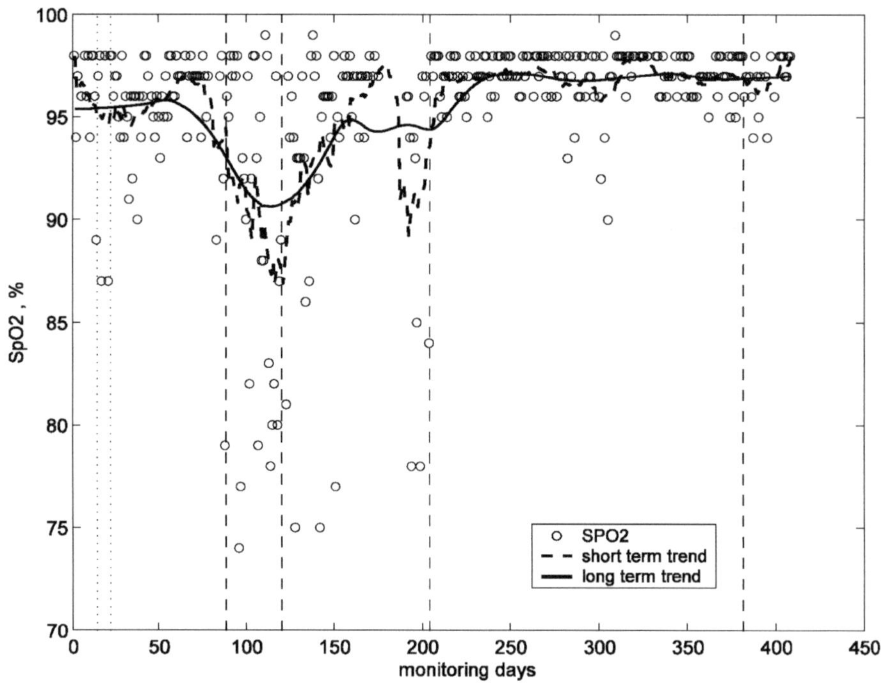

Figure 34.
Daily SpO_2 time-series data for patient with COPD [68].

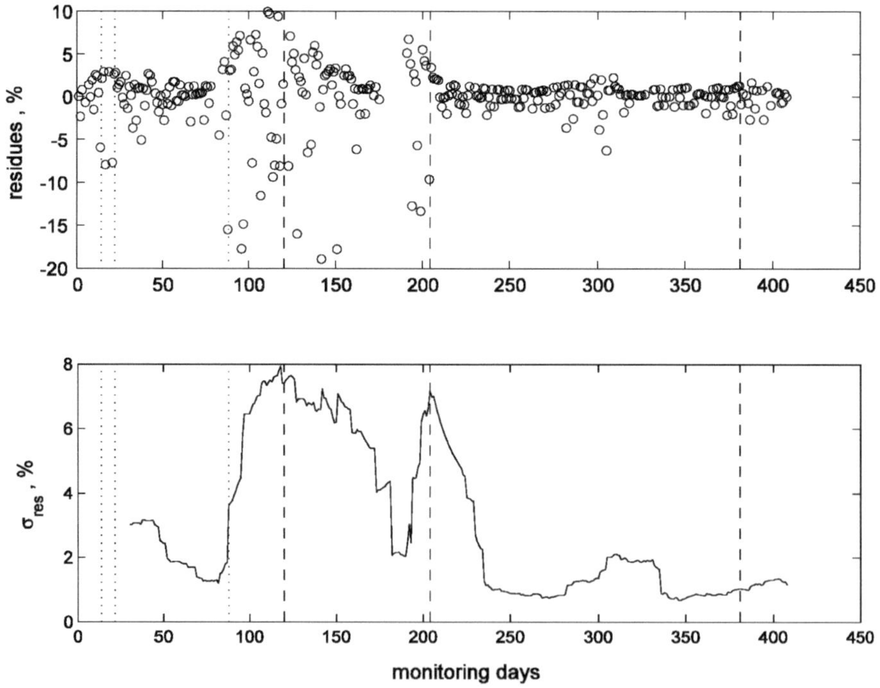

Figure 35.
Residuals (top) and estimates of standard deviation of residuals (bottom) [68].

7. Conclusion

Too often telehealth is seen as a panacea to resolve issues in a failing health service and is applied without consideration of the changes that must be made in order to integrate the telehealth into the existing service in terms of the technology, infrastructure, care pathways, new care services, management, support, training, new and changed roles, patient relationships, and professional relationships.

Telehealth is often promoted as being able to provide cost savings to the health service. Whilst reductions in length of stay, and possibly a reduction in the number of hospital admissions can be shown, resulting in notional savings, it is unlikely that the savings can be realised, as the hospital services will not be reduced. Most likely an organisation will be burdened with the additional costs for the technology and staff and the cost of providing services in the community. Or in cases where services have separate budgets, any saving in one service is not transferred as additional budget to the second. It is therefore essential that a holistic view be taken and all circumstances considered. For example, some organisations reimburse the costs of travel to the patient, and thus this would provide a realisable saving if the patient stays at home. In a single payer system, budget might be transferred, or made available to the organisation providing the telehealth service.

Alternatively a societal view may be taken. Telehealth can be seen as a solution to provide health services to communities and patients where otherwise it would not be available due to remoteness. Telehealth may also be considered to provide cost benefit to society by removing the need for costly travel for patient and relatives, and loss of earnings for time taken to travel and remain with the patient whilst in hospital.

Telehealth often suffers from poor design of the technology. Frequently devices are designed by enthusiastic young engineers to appeal to their imaginings of the needs of a patient; the system is built around the technology with which they are familiar, and does not relate to the needs of the actual user. At worst this means the technology is unusable with real patients (no broadband available, arthritic fingers cannot manipulate a smart phone, technology phobia), or is detested because it must be placed in a prominent position in the home and causes patients to be stigmatised. This problem also applies to procurement, when managers relate to the technology without understanding the needs of the patient; reminders may appear helpful but become irritating after many days of use. Telehealth should be simple and unobtrusive.

Moreover it must be recognised that telehealth is not a treatment, rather it is an approach to elicit relevant information from patients that may be used to support decision support and management. The effectiveness of outcome therefore relies on the services that use and act on that information. This may include telehealth supporting new approaches to deliver care. This may include using primary care and community to manage the patient, and using communication to support joint management and provide continuity of care, or establishing specialist services to manage the patient in the community. The approach adopted requires careful planning for its introduction.

However when implemented effectively, telehealth can confer significant benefit to the patient health, effectiveness of the clinician, and efficiency of the health service.

Author details

Malcolm Clarke
Ondokuz Mayis University, Samsun, Turkey

*Address all correspondence to: malcolm.clarke@omu.edu.tr

References

[1] Wootton R: Twenty years of telemedicine in chronic disease management – an evidence synthesis. J of Telemedicine and Telecare. 2012;18 (4):211-220. DOI: https://doi.org/10.1258/jtt.2012.120219.

[2] Bashshur RL, Howell JD, Krupinski EA, Harms KM, Bashshur N, Doarn CR: The Empirical Foundations of Telemedicine Interventions in Primary Care. Telemed J E Health. 2016; 22(5):342-375. DOI: 10.1089/tmj.2016.0045.

[3] Bensink M., Hailey D., Wootton R: A systematic review of successes and failures in home telehealth: preliminary results. Journal of Telemedicine and Telecare. 2006;12 (Suppl. 3): S3:8-16.

[4] Hays H, Carroll M, Ferguson S, Fore C, Horton M: The Success of Telehealth Care in the Indian Health Service. Virtual Mentor. 2014;16(12): 986-996. DOI: 10.1001/virtualmentor.2014.16.12.stas1-1412.

[5] Darkins A: The Growth of Telehealth Services in the Veterans Health Administration between 1994 and 2014: A Study in the Diffusion of Innovation. Telemedicine and e-Health. 2014;20(9): 761-8. DOI: https://doi.org/10.1089/tmj.2014.0143.

[6] VA's meteoric telehealth expansion poses new questions for the future. Access from: https://federalnewsnetwork.com/veterans-affairs/2021/04/vas-meteoric-telehealth-expansion-poses-new-questions-for-the-future/. [Accessed: 2021-10-01]

[7] Davis F.D: Perceived Usefulness, Perceived Ease of Use, and User Acceptance of Information Technology. MIS Quarterly. 1989;13(3):319-340.

[8] Davis F.D: User Acceptance of Information Technology System Characteristics, User Perceptions and Behavioral Impacts. International Journal of Man-Machine Studies. 1993; 38(3):475-487.

[9] Brewster L, Mountain G, Wessels B, Kelly C, Hawley M: Factors affecting frontline staff acceptance of telehealth technologies: a mixed-method systematic review. Journal of Advanced Nursing. 1993;70(1):21–33. DOI: 10.1111/jan.12196.

[10] Koivunen M, Saranto K: Nursing professionals' experiences of the facilitators and barriers to the use of telehealth applications: a systematic review of qualitative studies. Scand J Caring Sci. 2018;32:24–44.

[11] Sharma U, Clarke M: Nurses' and community support workers' experience of telehealth: a longitudinal case study. BMC health services research. 2014;14 (1):164.

[12] Sharma U, Barnett J, Clarke M: Understanding Innovation Deployment and Evaluation in Healthcare: The Triality Framework. In: Sun HY, editor. Management of Technological Innovation in Developing and Developed Countries. IntechOpen; 2012. p. 153-182. ISBN 9535103652. DOI: 10.5772/35671.

[13] Cimperman M, Brencic MM, Trkman P, de Leonni Stanonik M: Older Adults' Perceptions of Home Telehealth Services. Telemedicine and e-Health. 2013;19(10):786-90. DOI: https://doi.org/10.1089/tmj.2012.0272.

[14] Onyeachu P. The role of age and illness in the adoption of telehealth. Brunel University; 2016.

[15] Prochaska JO, Velicer WF: The transtheoretical model of health behavior change. Am J Health Promot. 1997;12(1):38-48. DOI: 10.4278/0890-1171-12.1.38.

[16] Ondiege B, Clarke M, Mapp G: Exploring a New Security Framework for Remote Patient Monitoring Devices. Computers. 2017;6(1):11; DOI: https://doi.org/10.3390/computers6010011.

[17] iPerf. Accessed from: http://iperf.fr. [Accessed: 2021-10-01]

[18] Mertens DM: Research and Evaluation in Education and Psychology, 3ed. Sage. 2010. ISBN 978-1-4129-7190-4.

[19] Alajlani M, Clarke M: Effect of Culture on Acceptance of Telemedicine in Middle Eastern Countries: Case study Jordan and Syria. Telemedicine and E-Health. 2013;19(4):305-311.

[20] Maucho L, Scott R, Mars M: Validation of an e-health readiness assessment framework for developing countries. BMC Health Services Research. 2020;20(1):575. DOI: 10.1186/s12913-020-05448-3.

[21] Hoppe KK, Williams M, Thomas N, et al: Telehealth with remote blood pressure monitoring for postpartum hypertension: A prospective single-cohort feasibility study. Pregnancy Hypertension. 2019;15:171–176. DOI: https://doi.org/10.1016/j.preghy.2018.12.007.

[22] IEEE 11073-20601-2019 - IEEE Health informatics–Personal health device communication - Part 20601: Application profile–Optimized Exchange Protocol. https://standards.ieee.org/standard/11073-20601-2019.html.

[23] Khan KS, Kunz R, Kleijnen, J, Antes, G: Five steps to conducting a systematic review. Journal of the Royal Society of Medicine. 2003;96(3):118–121. DOI: https://doi.org/10.1258/jrsm.96.3.118

[24] Garin O, Ferrer M, Pont A, Rué M, Kotzeva A, Wiklund I, Van Ganse E, Alonso J: Disease-specific health-related quality of life questionnaires for heart failure: a systematic review with meta-analyses. Qual Life Res. 2009;18(1):71-85. DOI: 10.1007/s11136-008-9416-4.

[25] Zhou Z, Zhou A, Zhao Y, Chen P: Evaluating the Clinical COPD Questionnaire: A systematic review. Respirology. 2017;22(2):251-262. DOI: 10.1111/resp.12970.

[26] Juniper EF, O'Byrne PM, Guyatt GH, Ferrie PJ, King DR: Development and validation of a questionnaire to measure asthma control. Eur Respir J. 1999;14:902–907.

[27] EQ5D. Available from: https://euroqol.org/ [Accessed: 2021-10-01]

[28] SF36. Accessed from: https://clinmedjournals.org/articles/jmdt/jmdt-2-023-figure-1.pdf. [Accessed: 2021-10-01]

[29] Gnani S, Ellis C: Trends in hospital admissions and case fatality due to heart failure in England 1990/91 to 1999/2000. Health Statistics Quarterly. 2001; 13:16-21.

[30] Arya A, Block M, Kautzner J, et al: Influence of Home Monitoring on the clinical status of heart failure patients: Design and rationale of the IN-TIME study. Eur J Heart Fail. 2008;10:1143-1148.

[31] Martínez A, Everss E, Rojo-Alvarez JL, Figal DP, García-Alberola A: A systematic review of the literature on home monitoring for patients with heart failure. J Telemed Telecare. 2006;12:234-241.

[32] Louis AA, Turner T, Gretton M, Baksh A, Cleland JG: A systematic review of telemonitoring for the management of heart failure. Eur J Heart Fail. 2003;5:583-590.

[33] Martínez A, Everss E, Rojo-Alvarez JL, Figal DP, García-Alberola A: A

systematic review of the literature on home monitoring for patients with heart failure. J Telemed Telecare. 2006;12: 234-241.

[34] Clark RA, Inglis SC, McAlister FA, Cleland JG, Stewart S: Telemonitoring or structured telephone support programmes for patients with chronic heart failure: systematic review and meta-analysis. BMJ. 2007;334:942.

[35] Roccaforte R, Demers C, Baldassarre F, Teo KK, Yusuf S: Effectiveness of comprehensive disease management programmes in improving clinical outcomes in heart failure patients. A meta-analysis. Eur J Heart Fail. 2005;7:1133-1144.

[36] Guallar-Castillón P, Banegas JR, Rodríguez-Artalejo F: The effectiveness of disease management programmes in reducing hospital re-admission in older patients with heart failure: a systematic review and meta-analysis of published reports. Eur Heart J 2004; 25: 1570-1595.

[37] Pinna GD, Maestri R, Andrews D, et al: Home telemonitoring of vital signs and cardiorespiratory signals in heart failure patients: system architecture and feasibility of the HHH model. Int J Cardiol. 2007;120:371-379.

[38] Gustafsson F, Arnold JM: Heart failure clinics and outpatient management: review of the evidence and call for quality assurance. Eur Heart J 2004; 25: 1596-1604.

[39] Clarke M, Shah A, Sharma U: Systematic Review of Studies on Telemonitoring of Patients with Congestive Heart Failure: A Meta-Analysis. Journal of Telemedicine and Telecare. 2011;17:7-14.

[40] Cleland J, Louis A, MD, Rigby A, Janssens U, Balk A: Noninvasive Home Telemonitoring for Patients With Heart Failure at High Risk of Recurrent Admission and Death The Trans-European Network–Home-Care Management System (TEN-HMS) Study. Journal of the American College of Cardiology. 2005;45: 1654–1664.

[41] Antonicelli R, Testarmata P, Spazzafumo L, Gagliardi C, Bilo G, Valentini M, Olivieri F, Parati G: Impact of telemonitoring at home on the management of elderly patients with congestive heart failure. Journal of Telemedicine and Telecare. 2008;14: 300–305.

[42] Balk A, Davidse W, Dommelen P, Klaassen E, Caliskan K, der Burgh P, Leenders C: Tele-guidance of chronic heart failure patients enhances knowledge about the disease. A multi-centre, randomised controlled study. European Journal of Heart Failure. 2008;10: 1136–1142.

[43] Woodend K, Sherrard H, Fraser M, Stuewe L, Cheung T, Struthers C: Telehome monitoring in patients with cardiac disease who are at high risk of readmission. Heart and Lung. 2008;37: 36–45.

[44] Wakefields B,Wrad M, Holman J, Roy A, Scherubel M, Burns T, Kienzle M, Rosenthal G: Evaluation of home telehealth following hospitalization for heart failure: A randomized trial. Telemedicine and e-health. 2008;14:753-761.

[45] Gokalp H, de Folter J, Verma V, Fursse J, Jones R, Clarke M: Integrated Telehealth and Telecare for Monitoring Frail Elderly with Chronic Disease. Telemedicine Journal and eHealth. 2018; 24(12):940-957. DOI: 10.1089/tmj.2017.0322.

[46] Lundell S, Holmer A, Rehn B, Nyberg A, Wadell K: Telehealthcare in COPD: A systematic review and meta-analysis on physical outcomes and dyspnea. Respiratory Medicine. 2015;

109(1):11-26. DOI: https://doi.org/10.1016/j.rmed.2014.10.008

[47] Jang S, Kim Y, Cho WK: A Systematic Review and Meta-Analysis of Telemonitoring Interventions on Severe COPD Exacerbations. Int. J. Environ. Res. Public Health. 2021;18: 6757-71. DOI: https://doi.org/10.3390/ijerph1813675

[48] Clarke M, Jones RW, Fursse J, Connelly-Brown N, Sharma U: Evaluation of the National Health Services (NHS) Direct Telehealth programme: cost-effectiveness analysis. Telemedicine Journal and eHealth. 2018; 24(1):67-77.

[49] Lee SWH, Chan CKY, Chua SS, et al: Comparative effectiveness of telemedicine strategies on type 2 diabetes management: A systematic review and network meta-analysis. Sci Rep. 2017;4:7(1):12680. DOI: https://doi.org/10.1038/s41598-017-12987-z.

[50] Nangrani N, Malabu U, Vangaveti V: Outcomes of Telehealth in the Management of Type 2 Diabetes—A Systematic Review and Meta-analysis of Randomised Controlled Trials. Diabetes. 2018;67(Supplement 1):. DOI: https://doi.org/10.2337/db18-1298-P.

[51] Kebede MM, Zeeb H, Peters M, Heise TL, Pischke CR: Effectiveness of Digital Interventions for Improving Glycemic Control in Persons with Poorly Controlled Type 2 Diabetes—A Systematic Review and Meta-regression Analysis. Diabetes Technol Ther. 2018;20(11):767-782. DOI: 10.1089/dia.2018.0216.

[52] De Groot J, Wu D, Flynn D, Robertson D, Grant G, Sun J: Efficacy of telemedicine on glycaemic control in patients with type 2 diabetes: A meta-analysis. World J Diabetes. 2021;12(2): 170-197. DOI: 10.4239/wjd.v12.i2.170.

[53] Gokalp H, Clarke M, Jones R, Fursse J, Sharma U: Whole Population Management of Patients with Diabetes. In: IEEE EMBS Special Topic Conference on Healthcare Innovation & Point-of-Care Technologies; October 2014; Seattle. 2014. DOI: 10.1109/HIC.2014.7038908.

[54] Huidi T, Kangambega P, Briatte C, Brunet-Houdard S, Retali G-R: Clinical Effectiveness of Telemedicine in Diabetes Mellitus: A Meta-analysis of 42 Randomized Controlled Trials. Telemedicine and e-Health. 2018;25(7): 569-583. DOI: 10.1089/tmj.2018.0128.

[55] Dexcom. Available from: https://www.dexcom.com/g6-cgm-system. [Accessed: 2021-10-01]

[56] Poolsup N, Suksomboon N, Kyaw AM: Systematic review and meta-analysis of the effectiveness of continuous glucose monitoring (CGM) on glucose control in diabetes. Diabetology & Metabolic Syndrome. 2013:5(1):39. DOI: 10.1186/1758-5996-5-39.

[57] Maiorino MI, Signoriello S, Maio A, et al: Effects of Continuous Glucose Monitoring on Metrics of Glycemic Control in Diabetes: A Systematic Review with Meta-analysis of Randomized Controlled Trials. Diabetes Care. 2020;43(5):1146-1156. DOI: https://doi.org/10.2337/dc19-1459.

[58] Choi WS, Choi JH, Oh J, Shin I-S, Yang J-S: Effects of Remote Monitoring of Blood Pressure in Management of Urban Hypertensive Patients: A Systematic Review and Meta-Analysis. Telemedicine and e-Health. 2020;26(6): 744-759. DOI: https://doi.org/10.1089/tmj.2019.0028.

[59] Rasekaba TM, Furler J, Blackberry I, Tacey M, Gray K, Lim K: Telemedicine interventions for gestational diabetes mellitus: A systematic review and meta-analysis. Diabetes Res Clin Pract. 2015; 110(1):1-9. DOI 10.1016/j.diabres.2015.07.007.

[60] Xie W, Dai P, Qin Y, Wu M, Yang B, Yu X: Effectiveness of telemedicine for pregnant women with gestational diabetes mellitus: an updated meta-analysis of 32 randomized controlled trials with trial sequential analysis. BMC Pregnancy Childbirth. 2020;20(1):198. DOI: 10.1186/s12884-020-02892-1.

[61] Fazal N, Webb A, Bangoura J, El Nasharty M: Telehealth: improving maternity services by modern technology. BMJ Open Qual. 2020;9(4):e000895. DOI: 10.1136/bmjoq-2019-000895.

[62] Nguyen E, Engle G, Subramanian S, Fryer K: Telemedicine for Prenatal Care: A Systematic Review. medRxiv 2021.05.14.21257232; DOI: https://doi.org/10.1101/2021.05.14.21257232.

[63] Clarke M, Bratan T, Kulkarni S, Jones R: The impact of remote patient monitoring in managing silent myocardial infarction in a residential home setting. Anadolu Kardiyoloji Dergisi. 2007;7(Suppl 1):186-188.

[64] Bratan T, Clarke M. Optimum Design of Remote Patient Monitoring Systems. In: International Conference of the IEEE Engineering in Medicine and Biology Society (EMBS 2006); 30 August - 3 September 2006; New York, NY. 2006. p. 6465-6468. DOI: 10.1109/IEMBS.2006.260729.

[65] Gokalp H, Clarke M: Monitoring activities of daily living of the elderly and the potential for its use in telecare and telehealth: A review. Telemedicine and E-Health, 2013;19(12):910-923.

[66] Clarke M, de Folter J, Verma V, Gokalp H: Interoperable End-to-End Remote Patient Monitoring Platform based on IEEE 11073 PHD and ZigBee Health Care Profile. Trans Biomedical Engineering. 2017;65(5):1014-1025. DOI:10.1109/TBME.2017.2732501.

[67] Connolly-Brown NE: A Better Way to Evaluate Remote Monitoring Programs in Chronic Disease Care: Receiver Operating Characteristic Analysis. Telemedicine and e-Health. 2014;20(12); 1143-1149. DOI: 10.1089/tmj.2014.0007.

[68] Clarke M, Gokalp H, Fursse J, Jones RW: Dynamic Threshold Analysis of Daily Oxygen Saturation for Improved Management of COPD Patients. IEEE J Biomed Health Inform. 2016;20(5):1352-1360. DOI: 10.1109/JBHI.2015.2464275.

Chapter 2

E-Health Applications for Smart and Pervasive Healthcare in Greece. What Can We Expect?

Sofia Voutsidou

Abstract

e-Health leads to the reshaping of the traditional ways of providing services by health professionals, aiming both at the rationalization of the expenses and the satisfaction of the patients-users of health services. Nevertheless, the key elements which prejudge its success are the measurable results, the guarantee of a broad consensus, as well as the leadership's commitment to implement it. In Greece, it is implemented within the European action eEurope 2005-eGovernment and the eEurope-i2010 programme. The application of e-Health in Greece is a national priority, for a number of reasons, such as the thousands of islands in the Greek archipelago which make the traditional form of medical care practically impossible. However, the economic crisis that broke out in Greece in 2009, as well as the arrival of waves of refugees in the country raised new issues in the development of the e-Health sector. This chapter analyses the institutional framework of e-Health in Greece. It also outlines the various technological, legal and organizational challenges that arise in the process of implementing e-Health in the pivots of effectiveness, efficiency, quality and equal accessibility. Finally, it develops a strategy for the future of e-Health in the Greek National Health System.

Keywords: e-Health, information and communication technologies, health services, telemedicine, accessibility

1. Introduction

The technological advances which occur at a rapid pace in the sectors of biomedicine, information technology and telecommunications, have already transformed fundamentally the entire spectrum of production and distribution of health services. The open e-government promotion leads in its turn, to the reshaping of the health sector, which is being called upon to respond to the contemporary challenges including the restriction of the expenses incurred, the effectiveness and simultaneous increase of the health services users' satisfaction [1, 2].

The Greek National Health System, especially after the prolonged period of economic crisis which it has experienced since 2009, faces up against accumulated problems in the citizen's relations with the services (responsiveness, quality and accessibility in the provided health services), having to solve a difficult equation. It's being required to balance and find the golden mean between the healthcare cost, which is constantly rising, since the destitute and uninsured citizens are multiplying, the population of Greece is aging, chronic and degenerative conditions are striking more and more people, while at the same time the refugees who arrive in the country amount to tens of thousands. On the other hand, the available system resources, both material and human, are constantly decreasing [3, 4]. Thus, inevitably, the need arises for healthcare in Greece to readjust to the new circumstances and utilize the digital technology so that hospital institutions will be decongested and healthcare expenditure limited [5, 6].

This paper will define the content of e-Health in accordance with the decisions of the World Health Organization and other international legal entities. It will then focus on how Greece implemented the specific decisions of international organizations. It will describe in detail the forms of e-Health adopted by the Greek National Health System, it will assess the benefits and the problems that have emerged from their implementation. Finally, it will discuss some of the challenges that Greece faces in the coming years in the context of the implementation of e-Health and highlight the role that the COVID-19 pandemic may play in accelerating them.

2. The concept of e-health

The term "e-Health" describes the utilization of modern technologies of Information Technology and telecommunications across the board of provided services by health professionals [7, 8]. In the framework of e-Health there are included programmes, systems and services which exceed the simple applications based on the Internet and are addressed both to health professionals and patients-users of health services, such as organized networks of health information, an electronic health record, an electronic health card, e-prescription, telemedicine, tele-counseling, tele-monitoring, personal portable communication systems, mobile phones and health portals. According to the World Health Organization [9] and the European Commission [10], e-Health refers to a wide range of products, systems and tools, which build their operation around the advanced information and communication technologies (ICT), aiming not only at the better management of health, but also the applied lifestyle on the whole. These online applications are addressed both to health professionals and patients-users and adopt a philosophy of a holistic approach, as they handle the prevention, diagnosis, treatment and later monitoring [11].

e-Health essentially comprises an emerging field in the intercept point of the scientific fields of medical informatics, public health and operational research. Its utilization focuses on the immediate, valid, qualitative and safe provision of health or healthcare services via the Internet and other available communication technologies. The desired effect is the transference of expertise and ensuring the smooth and unencumbered information flow, concerning not only healthcare, but also public health or preventive medicine [12].

At a global level, e-Health implementation is governed by the e-Health Resolution adopted by the 58th World Health Assembly in 2005 and aimed at better understanding [13] as well as its e-Health standardization and interoperability of World Health Organization [14], which stresses the need for standardization and interoperability of electronic applications, convergence of standards and their evaluation using common indicators, for comparable results. Furthermore, in 2012, the World Health Organization, in collaboration with the International Telecommunication Union (ITU), provided in the form of a manual the necessary guidelines to facilitate states in developing their national e-Health planning. This WHO-ITU National e-Health Strategy Toolkit [15] is a comprehensive operation plan and monitoring of e-Health applications and can be implemented by all countries wishing to develop or upgrade their national policy for e-Health, regardless of the level they are in today.

In Greece, its implementation was placed in the Greek framework of open government e-GIF (Electronic Government Interoperability Framework) and information online management, that was integrated in the Digital Agenda 2006–2013 (for the adjustment of services to the demands of the modern era), which was later readjusted in the framework of National Digital Strategy from 2016 to 2021 [16]. The Greek framework of open government specifies in essence the commands of the European action eEurope 2005-eGovernment and the programme eEurope-i2010, which divide the online provision of services in four axes: e-Government, e-Health, e-Learning and e-Business [17]. Towards the further propulsion of e-Health, the National Council of e-Health Management (NCHM) was established in 2015, which is headquartered in the Greek Ministry of Health.

3. Forms of e-health in Greece

e-Health does not only provide technological and procedural solutions to the needs of healthcare, but also reliable supportive applications, which are called upon to serve man, as the object and recipient of the health services provided. The tools that are employed in the context of e-Health promoting, are more effective, more user-friendly and more widely accepted both by the health professionals and the patients themselves. In e-Health applications there are included the electronic patient record, the electronic health card, e-prescription, development of telemonitoring and teleconsultation systems, as well as e-referral and electronic refund of medical expenses [18].

3.1 Electronic patient record

More specifically, the Electronic Patient Record or alternatively the Electronic Health Record comprises an individual electronic catalog, in which the medical data concerning the patient is registered and kept, so that its transference to any hospital institution or authorized doctor can be possible, aiming at a better diagnosis and limitation of medical mistakes [19, 20]. The same philosophy is served by using the electronic health card, so that an overview of its owner's health condition arises.

The electronic record includes data regarding the patient's medical history, such as their admission or readmission dates, their treatment duration, the results of laboratory and paraclinical tests conducted, the administered medicines and other treatment actions, information for the cost of the provided services, prior services offered as well as reports of acute cases, so as to constitute the patient's diagnosis basis and treatment approach, and at the same time the basis of epidemiological studies. In addition, it provides information of administrative, financial and statistical nature which is related to the respective hospital unit and the patient's demographic data (full name, VAT number, competent insurance institution, blood type), as well as quality control data [21].

The Electronic Health Record comprises an updated version of the Electronic Patient Record, as it aims at the continuous observation of its owner's health and not exclusively during their treatment period. In contrast with handwritten records, it ensures the preservation of the registered data (health data, laboratory results, medical instructions, imaging records, bio-signal records), and their endurance through time, it allows their holistic management while providing interconnection capacity via applications of data transmission. This way, it facilitates the provision of medical consultation remotely, simultaneously enabling the electronic prescription. It also contributes to the timely and correct illness diagnosis, the right observation of patients, the elimination of multiple registrations, the operational cost reduction (e.g. avoidance of pointless examinations, facilitation of payment, distribution of resources connected to the diagnosis and treatment), and at the same time it creates a constantly developing "electronic library" which is also compatible with research purposes [22–24].

Since the data which is included in the patient's medical record, fall within the most sensitive personal information (main illness, history of present illness, allergies and medicines, medical history, family history, social history, occupational history, sexual history, addiction to use of drug, smoke and other substances), every aspect of their safety, confidentiality and protection must be ensured substantially [25, 26]. In the last few years, the Citizen Health Record has been promoted in Europe, which corresponds more thoroughly to the contemporary vision of the globalized citizen, as far his expectations from the health services are concerned. It is an improved version which fully covers the digital recording and preservation of the contents of the electronic medical record and simultaneously deals successfully with the problems that arise from its electronic nature [27].

In Greece, the creation of a National Medical Record is being promoted, in order that all the necessary information regarding a citizen's health condition (hospital treatments, medical opinions, imaging and laboratory examinations, prescriptions, etc.) will accompany them from now on [28]. The efficiency of this modern digital tool will be bidirectional. On the one hand, it will guide and facilitate the citizen in their contact with the National Health System (e.g. through the application myHealth, the appointment making will be conducted digitally, as well as the system navigation). Nonetheless, at the same time it will comprise a "portal" of access to their data for the treating doctors, so that they have the full medical history available, thus abolishing the printed records. The first step has been taken with the activation of the Individual Electronic Health Record. In the next stage, there is the provision of its further reinforcement and its gradual disengagement from the Family Doctor through legislative interventions [29]. As the General Secretary of the Ministry of Health stated, in the electronic record there will be included the patient's biochemistry and blood tests, as well as the main clinical documents of the hospitals that concern them [30].

The formation process of the Electronic Patient Record is advancing at a satisfactory pace. It is noteworthy that the non-profit Public Company under the name "Electronic Government of Social Insurance" (IDIKA P.C.), which undertook the implementation of the project, was awarded an international distinction at the awards ceremony of the World Information Technology and Services Association "WITSA Global ICT Excellence Awards 2019" that took place in the context of the World Congress on Information Technology, on October 8th, 2019 in Erevan, Armenia. The project of the Electronic Health Record (EHR) was distinguished as Merit Winner in the category "Innovative eHealth Solutions" [31].

It should also be pointed out that the pandemic of COVID-19 gave a new impetus to the formation process of the electronic record in Greece. In particular, in April 2020, there was enforced by the Greek Ministry of Health and the Ministry of Digital Government the Electronic COVID-19 Patients Register. In this way, the contact of patients suffering from COVID-19 with their treating doctors was simplified, especially in the sectors of tele-consultation and both intangible and remote prescription. What is more, it should be highlighted that based on the Greek and European Law, the patients' personal data are protected, as health services have at their disposal merely the information which is helpful for the handling of the pandemic [32].

3.2 Electronic prescription

Furthermore, the adoption and application of electronic programmes in the field of pharmaceutical policy, such as the medicine list and the electronic prescription, contributes crucially to the rational management of the provided pharmaceutical services, ensuring the appropriate and more economical care with a simultaneous minimization of expenses [33]. The uniform electronic medicine list includes the approved available pharmaceutical preparations, their cost and the amount of their provided for compensation.

Despite the fact that this specific list mainly comprises a clinical tool, facilitating the doctors' e-prescription substantially, it also assists by its central management, the significant restriction of pharmaceutical expenditure, in combination with the promoted policy of generic medicine selection (i.e. the copies of pharmaceutical preparations), instead of the original ones which are more expensive due to the patent they possess [34, 35]. Additionally, both the electronic entries of the prescriptions on the part of the doctors with the help of personalized passwords and the obligatory prescription based on the active substance and not the commercial name of the preparation, allows the wider administration of the more economical generic medicines and the electronic monitoring of medical prescription behavior in real time [36, 37].

During the COVID-19 pandemic, it became clear that the utilization of digital technologies is the only safe way in order for the patients to gain access to the health system. Thus, in the summer of 2020, the intangible electronic medicine prescription was established by law in Greece (L. 4704/2020). Both the intangible prescription and the intangible referral are transferred now exclusively using electronic means to the Primary Healthcare System. The patients log in there and state that they wish to receive their medicine prescription electronically, either through a message (SMS) on their mobile phone or via an email to their email address. In the fulfillment of the intangible electronic prescription, the printed form of the doctor's medicine prescription is not submitted to the chemist. The chemist retrieves the intangible electronic prescription by entering in the Electronic Prescription System the prescription barcode or the patient's Social Security Registration Number (SSRN) [38].

3.3 National Network of telemedicine (NNTM)

The potential that new technologies offer is expanded in the field of telemedicine, tele-monitoring and teleconsultation, as well. The utilization of telemedicine and telecare, which means the remote support or provision of health services by specialized and suitably trained health professionals to that purpose, goes a long way towards dealing in a timely manner with situations that could turn out to be a health hazard. Therefore, it is about technical knowledge transfer instead of patient transfer. Its major significance lies in the fact that it provides the possibility of remote support for patient management at the regional health facilities by general medicine practitioners.

In Greece, a mainly insular country which is divided in seven health regions, there has been materialized a National Network of Telemedicine since 2016, headquartered in the country's 2nd Regional Health Authority to which the large port of Piraeus and the Aegean islands belong. The same year, NNTM won the award of Business I.T. Excellence Gold (BITE) for its output, which is awarded in cases where technological innovation coincides with business excellence. The Network of Telemedicine is based on the Public Data Network of OTE "INTERCONNECTION" and it includes 43 telemedicine units. Those are based on 12 regional and central hospitals, as well as 30 centers of the Aegean islands, including the border islands of Astypalaia, Icaria, Kalymnos, Ios, Kasos, Kastellorizo. Lastly, there is a telemedicine unit in the center of operations of the Greek Ministry of Health [39].

The National Telemedicine Center is bound to be expanded to 22 additional islands of the Northern and South Aegean, covering the healthcare needs of 52 islands on the whole, with 71 telemedicine units and 90 patient monitoring systems at home [40]. This way, there is provided an equal access of the island regions patients to the services of the National Health System. At the same time, the pointless transfers and evacuations by air are limited, simultaneously relieving the hospitals Out-patient Clinics.

Every telemedicine unit consists of a specially configured chamber, a camera, a screen and appropriate medical instruments that broadcast the indications of examinations live at hospitals of Athens and Piraeus. In this effort towards not only the provision of specialized health services, but also the guidance and education of the regional health professional in the Aegean islands which are isolated from the major urban centers, 270 health professionals participate, among whom 67 doctors-consultants from 27 different specialties (Psychiatry, Child-Psychiatry, Pediatrics, Surgery, Pediatric Surgery, Breast Surgery, Orthopedics, Pathology, Bio-pathology, Pathologic Oncology, Cardiology, Dermatology, Medical Imaging, Dentistry, Pulmonology, Obstetrics-Gynecology, Chest Surgery, Plastic Surgery, Nuclear Medicine, Ophthalmology, Rheumatology, Gastroenterology, Endocrinology, Nephrology, Urology, Critical Care Specialist, Emergency Unit Specialist) [39]. The examinations categories which are mainly requested are child-psychiatric, endocrinologic, diabeteologic, psychiatric and oncologic [40]. In a country such as Greece, which has over 90 islands, the telemedicine network is estimated to serve the needs of more than 320,000 permanent residents and a fairly large number of visitors each year [41].

According to the information available, there were held more than 4,500 appointments of specialized health services provision in regular and emergency incidents in Aegean islands of the Greek-Turkish border through the NNTM. At the same time, actions of prevention and promotion of oral hygiene were conducted to children aged 6–12 in Chios (Pyrgi, Kalamoti), in Oinousses and Icaria's Fournoi, as well as an action of prevention aimed at children and adolescents of the border island of Ios about mental health issues. Furthermore, continuous education of the health professionals who staff the insular health units is carried out, the main bodies being the University General Hospital "Atticon" and the General Nikaia Hospital "Agios Panteleemon". It is interesting that over 300 educational seminars have been materialized to date. Alongside, in the education context of the general population, junior high and high school students of Lesbos island (Antissa) were educated on Basic Life Support (BLS) and the use of an automatic external defibrillator.

Moreover, the telemedicine network is used for administrative support, with frequent video-conferences (approximately 70,000 teleconferences were carried out up to November 2020) for the further familiarization with the use of the system and primarily for the change of philosophy of the employees in the sector of health and the adoption of the operation of NNTM on everyday practice. What is especially important is the free-of-charge provision of tele-interpreting for the facilitation of hospital institutions and Health Centers in the handling of incidents where there is no common communication language between the patient and the health professionals. As far as the future goals of NNTM are concerned, they include the integration of emergency incidents in the hospital shifts, in order to achieve a 24-hour coverage of the Aegean islands, at least concerning cardiologic and pediatric incidents.

3.4 Patient tele-monitoring

An advancement of telemedicine is the provision of health services at home, which supports tele-monitoring and tele-management of patients in their own premises. The health professionals, who provide care remotely, can diagnose X-rays, receive a medical history from patients, assess laboratory findings and suggest courses of treatment. Electronic recording devices are used, which send the data to the treating doctor, and then he/she on his/her part, having all the necessary documentation, consults the patient-user comprehensively. The system under discussion addresses mostly patients with heart disease, pulmonary disease, hypertension and diabetes, who require long-term monitoring. Nevertheless, there is also the possibility to utilize it in the monitoring of patients having different treatment needs, such as post-operative or psychiatric patients [42].

Greece has also demonstrated significant progress in the sector of patient telemonitoring in the last few years. More specifically, the following programmes are being carried out:

3.4.1 Telecare programme renewing health

The programme was applied for the first time at 2014 in the area of Thessaly, in Central Greece, granting monitoring remote services to patients with chronic conditions, in particular to patients with type 2 diabetes, cardiovascular disease and obstructive pulmonary disease. It is noteworthy that in the cases of the patients suffering from diabetes and cardiovascular failure, there were noted positive clinical results as far as intervention via tele-monitoring is concerned. However, at the same time various problems arose, such as the slow pace of adoption of technological innovations in healthcare, the complexity of the institutional framework, the lack of compensation models, as well as the lack of interoperability in telemedicine infrastructure. The Greek Ministry of Health is making an effort to resolve all those problems [43].

3.4.2 SmartCare programme

It's a European programme in which the Greek Municipalities of Palaio Faliro, Alimos and Agios Dimitrios participated. The project was related with the development and incorporation of technologies in the existing care structures for the independent living of patients and the elderly at home (home platforms). The programme provided various services, such as observation of the patients' physiological, environmental and behavioral parameters, self-care functions, management of the patients' medication, prevention of falls and accidents and practice of the patients' cognitive functions [43].

3.4.3 United4Health programme

In the programme United for Health, there were overall 33 participants from all Europe as well as international organizations from the sector of electronic health. Greece took part through the 5th Regional Health Authority of Thessaly and Continental Greece, as well as via the "Cities NET S.A." (Larissa, Ioannina, Volos, Lamia, Kozani, Katerini, Veria, Karditsa, Trikala and Grevena) after being granted permission from the competent Ministries. The programme had a duration of 3 years and a total budget of 10,151,56 Euros for all Europe, while it was cofounded by the European Committee. In the context of the programme, there were selected patients suffering from chronic diseases (such as diabetes mellitus for the case of the pilot in Greece) by the treating doctors with the criteria of the need for intensive home monitoring and adjustment of medication [44]. There were utilized some conclusions from the Renewing Health Telecare Programme in Central Greece and there were organized telecare services of an out-patient clinic in actual conditions. The study conclusions demonstrated that the clinical efficacy of telecare for diabetes mellitus patients is feasible, depending on the service per National Health System, though [43].

3.5 Video-communication stations for the deaf and hearing-impaired

The National Institution for Deaf People of Greece, since March of 2019, began to develop a new form of service for people with hearing/impaired hearing problems with the aid of technology (Relay Service). The referred to service is of a 24-hour cycle. People with hearing/impaired hearing problems can make use of the electronic appliance on their mobile phone or on an electronic computer of any kind and contact a special interpreter via video call. By using the programme, the improvement of communication and service of the deaf and hearing-impaired is achieved, as the transmission of information to health professionals is facilitated. By extension, the users are able to receive equally quality health services at the levels of prevention, diagnosis, treatment, hospital treatment, rehabilitation and support in administrative services.

In the framework of social support for the disabled, the specific initiative was adopted by the Ministry of Health in Greece, anticipating inequality decrease and equal access to social communication commodities for all citizens. With a document from the Administration of Primary Healthcare of the Greek Ministry of Health (Γ1γ/ΓΦ.20.ΣΤ/ΓΠ. 66393/26.10.2020), it was requested by all structures and services of healthcare provision, both of the public (Hospitals, Health Centers, Centers of Mental Health and other supervised bodies of the Ministry of Health) and the private sector (private clinics, private practices, dental practices, group practices, laboratories, units of daily treatment) to accept and utilize the recommended authorized way of communication through the programme of Relay Service in order to accommodate the deaf and hearing-impaired, as well as for the provision of services in which their physical presence is not required [45].

The first video-communication station for the deaf and hearing-impaired in Greece operated in July 2020 at the “Laikon” General Hospital of Attica. According to the national plan, 30 stations of video-communication for the deaf and hearing-impaired are expected to operate for a trial period of one (1) year both in hospitals and other public services and bodies of common interest in Greece, for instance Local Authorities, Regions, Airports and the Underground [46].

The example of the “Laikon” General Hospital of Attica was followed, in October 2020, by the 4th Macedonia and Thrace Regional Health Authority, which announced the operation initiation of three (3) video-communication stations for the deaf and hearing-impaired at the AHEPA University General Hospital, the Alexandroupoli University General Hospital and at the 25th Martiou Health Center in Thessaloniki [47].

3.6 Mobile health (m-health)

One of the subdivisions of e-Health is the exploitation of mobile phones, mobile Health (m-Health). The cellular phone is proved to be the handiest tool nowadays, as it has evolved into a personal object that the majority of the population uses and does not part with. It can be recruited in the context of e-Health in a variety of ways: notification of the patient about the taking of their medication through automatized messages, their scheduled appointments or reminders to pregnant women either about different stages of pregnancy or advice when they cope with an unusual condition [48–50].

In Greece, mobile Health was used extensively during the COVID-19 pandemic. In this context, a special hotline of psychosocial support operated in Greece (10306) by the National Public Health Organization. The hotline service was offered under the supervision of the Medical School of the National and Kapodistrian Athens University [51].

4. The contribution of e-health to smart and pervasive healthcare. Challenges for Greece in formulating a national strategy for the future of e-health

e-Health certainly does not constitute the "magic solution" for the existing health system's various problems in infrastructure, staffing, organization and resources. However, it can significantly enable the successful dealing with its chief function issues, optimizing the provided services of Primary Healthcare. In particular, e-Health ensures fast, valid, reliable and directly accessible medical information for everyone, which covers not only topics of general interest, but also specific issues that cope with specific needs. By the exploitation of the possibilities it grants, the prompt and correct diagnosis of diseases becomes feasible, as well as the regular monitoring of patients and the remote provision of medical consultation, with an emphasis on preventive medicine. It also facilitates both the medical care of people who reside in isolated areas and individualized medical healthcare in combination with patients' safety [52].

The applications of e-Health contribute to the correct diagnosis, with the assistance of non-invasive systems that base their function on imaging. Thus, the sector of Primary Healthcare provision is re-determined and expanded, regionally and temporally, as well as with regard to the speediness, utilization easiness, availability, operability, possibilities of control and cost reduction, the degree of participation and awareness, combined with the improvement of service of the patients-users [53].

By utilizing e-Health extensively, the exchange of data is facilitated, while at the same time, standardized forms of communication are now created between health professionals. Primarily, however, a new status is given to the interaction and mutual cooperation of the doctor with the patient, which must, nonetheless, be governed by honesty, trustworthiness and confidentiality [54].

e-Health is a key component that the European Union also emphasizes in the setting of Europe 2020 targets [10]. As of 2011, the European Commission's Implementing Decision of 22 December laying down the rules for the establishment, management and operation of the network of national authorities responsible for e-Health (Decision 2011/890/EU) entered into force. The following year, the European Commission, through the Directorate-General for Health of the European Union, adopted common rules of procedure for the implementation of the e-Health network in European countries, aiming at interoperability and uniform evaluation [12]. Concerning the Member States of the European Union, according to a press release issued by the European Commission on the extent of e-Health in Europe, the use of e-Health systems has been generalized in most European countries. The pioneers are: Denmark, the Netherlands, Great Britain, Estonia, Sweden, Finland and Germany. More specifically, the countries that perform best in the implementation of e-Health in hospitals are Denmark (66%), Estonia (63%) and closely followed by Sweden and Finland (62%). In the digitization of medical files the best performance has been made by the Netherlands (83.2%), followed by Denmark (80.6%) and Great Britain (80.5%), while Estonia stands out (100%) in e-prescription followed by Croatia (99%) and Sweden (97%) [55].

In 2015, the top ten European States in e-Health applications between doctors and patients were as follows: Denmark, Finland, Spain, the Netherlands, Sweden, Estonia, Croatia, Portugal, Germany and France. The e-Health applications evaluated included physicians' ability to diagnose and prescribe electronically, the ability of health professionals to exchange data, make appointments with patients, and communicate with care providers, medical surveillance, patients' electronic information about their health and the ability to obtain valid information via the Internet [56].

In Greece, e-Health has experienced a rapid development in the last two decades. As contradictory as it may sound, the economic crisis following 2019 became an opportunity for the country to proceed to extensive changes in the National Health System. That was necessary since health expenditure had to be significantly reduced. In this context, e-Health applications were deemed very effective so that the country could secure resources for the repayment of foreign loans. According to the European Union data, per capita expenditure in the health sector in Greece in 2009 amounted to 2,287 Euros. That amount decreased to 1,650 Euros in 2015 [57], a sum which is 45% lower than the European Union average [58].

An additional pressure to the National Health System was given by the thousands of refugees who arrived in the country in the last few years. According to the data, only in the year of 2015, Greece in collaboration with NPO, provided medical care to approximately 870,000 refugees. The available data shows that, from the e-Health sectors, e-prescription has proved to be an essential factor towards expenditure restriction. It is estimated that in the time period 2009–2014, 3 billion Euros were saved thanks to intangible prescription [59].

The last pandemic of COVID-19 is expected to contribute even more towards the reinforcement of e-Health. In various countries, there have already been made and are currently functioning applications of tracking of contacts for cell phones. The said applications are installed voluntarily and, by using the Bluetooth technology, warn the users who were very close to a person affected by the virus for a period of time. In this way, it is possible to control the expansion of the infection more easily. Nonetheless, it is vital that the privacy and personal information of the users be protected, with the commitment from the national authorities that they will not make use of them and that they will deactivate the respective applications as soon as the pandemic has been overcome [60].

However, the way towards the direction of a smart and pervasive healthcare is still long both for Greece and the rest of the world. The only thing certain is that it is a one-way street. In our era, the era of the Fourth Industrial Revolution, e-Health is expected to experience an exponential growth in the years to come.

Unfortunately, in the case of Greece there are still no reliable financial data on the cost of implementing e-Health programmes and the benefits of their implementation. This is a significant lag in relation to the European reality, which is undoubtedly an obstacle on the further promotion of e-Health in Greece. The only reliable data that has been able to be found are based on research by the Association of Greek Industries which include as good practice the application of the National Network of Telemedicine in the remote Greek islands as well as the case of a public hospital, which is included in smart hospitals, i.e. those hospitals that have largely implemented the digitization of their services [61].

5. Conclusions

e-Health can yield significant benefits to the society as a whole, contributing conspicuously to the accessibility and quality of the provided health services to the citizens who are in need of them. Furthermore, it helps towards the development of a National Health System with an anthropocentric orientation, founded on the viability of the health field, with the spreading of correct practices and the optimal exploitation of the available resources, both material and human. Moreover, e-Health is bound to increase the effectiveness and efficiency of the services provided by health professionals, thus contributing to the rationalization and reduction of expenditure.

The promotion of e-Health renders possible the provision of better care to more patients, releasing the institutional resources (of Hospitals, Clinics, Health Centers,

Regional Surgeries) and limiting healthcare expenses. The new technologies provide various possibilities, readjusting the provided healthcare forms, depending on the individualized needs and expectations of every patient. Geographical distances are nullified and the provision range of health services is expanded, granting equal access even to residents of removed from the urban centers areas. This way, the citizens' feeling of their equal participation to the public commodities is consolidated, particularly to those who live in remote and isolated areas.

There are certainly several issues which must be resolved so as for e-Health to be reinforced. It is essential that all bodies concerned, and especially Leadership, realize the value and the advantages which derive from its utilization. It is also necessary that e-Health applications be more user-friendly. Above all, though, there must be ensured the confidentiality of the transmitted information and the patients' personal data. Only in this way will everybody understand that e-Health can really contribute towards the direction of a smart and pervasive healthcare.

In the case of Greece, it is necessary to have measurable results that prove in practice the benefits of implementing smart and pervasive healthcare. In addition, the Greek National Health System needs to adopt good practices, which are already successfully applied in other European countries, such as Denmark, Estonia and Finland.

Conflict of interest

The author declares no conflict of interest.

Author details

Sofia Voutsidou
Central Services, 4th Regional Health Authority Macedonia and Thrace,
Thessaloniki, Greece

*Address all correspondence to: svoutsidou@gmail.com

References

[1] Buse K, Drager N, Fustukian S, Lee K. Globalization and health policy: trends and opportunities. In: Lee K, Buse K, Fustukian S, editors. Health policy in a globalising world. Cambridge: Cambridge University Press; 2002. pp. 251-280.

[2] Lenk K, Traunmuller R. Broadening the Concept of Electronic Government. In: Prins JEJ, editor. Designing e-Government. 2nd ed. Amsterdam: Kluwer Law International; 2001. pp. 63-74.

[3] Kentikelenis A, Karanikolos M, Papanicolas I, Basu S, Mckee M, Stuckler D. Health effects of financial crisis: omens of a Greek tragedy. The Lancet. 2011; 378: 1457-1468. DOI: 10.1016/S0140-6736(11)61556-0.

[4] Chalkia V, Varaklioti A. Health and social protection expenditure in Greece and the EU-member states. Archives of Hellenic Medicine. 2015; 32: 546-555.

[5] Tsounis A, Sarafis P. Qualitive electronic management of information in health services as an implement of ensuring of total quality. Interscientific Health Care. 2012; 4:91-97.

[6] Liaropoulos L. Organization of Health Services and Systems. Athens: Beta Publications; 2007. 199-202 pp.

[7] Callens S, Cierkens K. Legal Aspects of E-HEALTH. In: De Clercq E, De Moor G, Bellon J, Foulon M, Van der Lei J, editors. Collaborative Patient Centred eHealth. Proceedings of the HIT@HealthCare 2008 joint event: 25th MIC Congress, 3rd International Congress Sixi, Special ISV-NVKVV Event, 8th Belgian eHealth Symposium. Amsterdam: IOS Press; 2008. pp. 47-56.

[8] Kluge EH. e-Health Promises and Challenges: Some Ethical Considerations. In: Borycki EM, Bartle-Clar JA, Househ MS, Kuziemsky CE, Schraa EG, editors. International Perspectives in Health Informatics. Amsterdam: IOS Press; 2011. pp. 148-153.

[9] World Health Organization. Global Observatory for eHealth [Internet]. 2016. Global diffusion of eHealth: Making universal health coverage achievable. Available from: https://apps.who.int/iris/bitstream/handle/10665/252529/9789241511780-eng.pdf;jsessionid=1976C9C262C24A61C9B551224A4E11B7?sequence=1 [Accessed: 2020-10-20].

[10] European Commission. Public Health, eHealth: Digital Health and Care [Internet]. 2015. Available from: http://ec.europa.eu/health/ehealth/policy/index_en.htm [Accessed: 2020-10-25].

[11] Ball MJ, Lillis J. E-health: transforming the physician/patient relationship. International Journal of Medical Informatics. 2001; 61:1-10. DOI: 10.1016/s1386-5056(00)00130-1.

[12] European Commission. eHealth Action Plan 2012-2020: Innovative healthcare for the 21st century [Internet]. 2012. Available from: http://ec.europa.eu/digital-agenda/en/news/ehealth-action-plan-2012-2020-innovative-healthcare-21st-century [Accessed: 2020-10-23].

[13] World Health Organization. 58th World Health Assembly [Internet]. 2005. Available from: https://apps.who.int/gb/ebwha/pdf_files/WHA58-REC1/english/A58_2005_REC1-en.pdf [Accessed: 2020-10-20].

[14] World Health Organization. eHealth standardization and interoperability [Internet]. 2013, Available from: https://apps.who.int/iris/bitstream/handle/10665/78878/B132_R8-en.pdf?sequence=1&isAllowed=y [Accessed: 2020-11-12].

[15] WHO-ITU. National eHealth Strategy Toolkit [Internet]. 2012. Available from: https://www.itu.int/dms_pub/itu-d/opb/str/D-STRE_HEALTH.05-2012-PDF-E.pdf [Accessed: 2020-10-10].

[16] Greek Ministry of Digital Policy, Telecommunications and Information. National Digital Strategy 2016-2021 [Internet]. 2016. Available from: http://www.opengov.gr/digitalandbrief/wp-content/uploads/downloads/2016/11/digital_strategy.pdf [Accessed: 2020-10-17].

[17] Alexopoulos Ch. Interoperability of Information Systems. Field Theoretical Analysis and Documentation [thesis]. Karlovasi: Aegean University; 2011.

[18] European Commission. Public health, eHealth: Digital health and care [Internet]. 2015. Available from: http://ec.europa.eu/health/ehealth/policy/index_en.html [Accessed: 2020-10-12].

[19] Dillon TW. Nursing Attitudes and Images of Electronic Patient Record Systems. Computers Informatics Nursing. 2005; 23:139-145. DOI: 10.1097/00024665-200505000-00009.

[20] Oborn E, Barrett M, Davidson E. Unity in Diversity: Electronic Patient Record Use in Multidisciplinary Practice. Information Systems Research. 2011; 22:419-484. DOI: 10.2307/23015594.

[21] Michel-Verkerke MB, Stegwee RA, Spil TA. The six P's of the next step in electronic patient records in the Netherlands. Health Policy and Technology. 2015; 4:137-143. DOI: 10.1016/j.hlpt.2015.02.011.

[22] Roussel F, Darmoni SJ, Thirion B. Cost effectiveness of a medical digital library. Medical Informatics and the Internet in Medicine. 2001; 26:325-330. DOI: 10.1080/14639230110097824.

[23] Uslu AM, Stausberg J. Value of the electronic patient record: an analysis of the literature. Journal of Biomedical Informatics. 2008; 41:675-682. DOI: 10.1016/j.jbi.2008.02.001.

[24] Ventres WB, Frankel RM. Patient-centered Care and Electronic Health Records: It's Still About the Relationship. Family Medicine. 2010; 42:364-366. DOI: 10.1080/10401334.2013.827981.

[25] Zeng X, Reynolds R, Sharp M. Redefining the Roles of Health Information Management Professionals in Health Information Technology. Online Research Journal Perspectives in Health Information Management. 2009; 6:1f.

[26] Mathai N, Shiratudin MF, Sohel F. Electronic Health Record Management: Expectations, Issues and Challenges. Journal of Health and Medical Informatics. 2017; 8:1-5. DOI: 10.4172/2157-7420.1000265.

[27] European Commission. Synopsis Report. Consultation: Transformation Health and Care in the Digital Single Market [Internet]. 2018. Available from: https://ec.europa.eu/health/sites/health/files/ehealth/docs/2018_consultation_dsm_en.pdf [Accessed: 2020-10-17].

[28] Greek Ministry of Digital Policy, Telecommunications and Information. National Digital Strategy Operational Progress Report 2016-2021 [Internet]. 2016. Available from: http://www.ictplus.gr/files/PDF%20FILES/DIGITAL_STRATEGY_2016_2021.pdf [Accessed: 2020-11-14].

[29] To Vima. Health is dynamically entering the digital age [Internet]. 2020. Available from: https://www.tovima.gr/2020/06/04/society/i-ygeia-mpainei-dynamika-stin-psifiaki-epoxi [Accessed: 2020-10-25].

[30] Business Daily. The National Health File is implemented before the end of

the year [Internet]. 2020. Available from: https://www.businessdaily.gr/koinonia/21917_mpainei-se-efarmogi-prin-telos-toy-etoys-o-ethnikos-fakelos-ygeias [Accessed: 2020-10-29].

[31] Citizen Guide. Electronic Health Record (EHR) for every Citizen [Internet]. 2019. Available from: http://www.odigostoupoliti.eu/ilektronikos-fakelos-ygeias-ify-gia-kathe-politi/ [Accessed: 2020-11-12].

[32] Greek Ministry of Health. Electronic Patient Register COVID-19 [Internet]. 2020. Available from: https://covid19.gov.gr/ilektroniko-mitroo-asthenon-covid-19/ [Accessed: 2020-10-27].

[33] Vandoros S, Stargardt T. Reforms in the Greek pharmaceutical market during the financial crisis. Health Policy. 2013; 109:1-6. DOI: 10.1016/j.healthpol.2012.08.016.

[34] Kontodimopoulos N, Kastanioti C, Thireos E, Karanikas H, Polyzos N. The contribution of generic substitution to rationalizing pharmaceutical expenditure in Greek public hospitals under recent economic crisis. Journal of Pharmaceutical Health Services Research. 2013; 4:211-216. DOI: 10.1111/jphs.12032.

[35] Economou Ch, Kaitelidou D, Kentikelenis A, Sissouras A, Maresso A. Case Study. The impact of the financial crisis on the health system and health in Greece. World Health Organization-European Observatory on Health Systems and Policies [Internet]. 2014. Available from: http://www.euro.who.int/__data/assets/pdf_file/0007/266380/The-impact-of-the-financial-crisis-on-the-health-system-and-health-in-Greece.pdf [Accessed: 2020-10-18].

[36] Mossialos E, Allin S, Davaki K. Analysing the Greek health system: a tale of fragmentation and inertia. Health Economics. 2005; 14:S151-S168. DOI: 10.1002/hec.1033.

[37] Xanthopoulou S, Katsaliaki K. Evaluation of generic drug use in the Greek market during the financial crisis. Archives of Hellenic Medicine. 2016; 33:583-595.

[38] Greek Ministry of Health. Intangible prescription [Internet]. 2020. Available from: https://www.gov.gr/ipiresies/ugeia-kai-pronoia/phakelos-ugeias/aule-suntagographese [Accessed: 2020-10-09].

[39] 2nd Regional Health Authority Piraeus and Aegean. Telemedicine [Internet]. 2016. Available from: http://www.2dype.gr/tileiatriki [Accessed: 2020-10-23].

[40] Protagon.gr. Expansion of the National Telemedicine Network to another 22 Aegean islands [Internet]. 2020. Available from: https://www.protagon.gr/themata/epektasi-tou-ethnikou-diktyou-tileiatrikis-se-akomi-22-nisia-tou-aigaiou-44342094422 [Accessed: 2020-11-14].

[41] European Parliament-Workshop STOA (Science and Technology Options Assessment). eHealth in Europe: Reality and challenges ahead. Participants' booklet [Internet]. 2015. Available from: www.europarl.europa.eu/cmsdata/149015/Booklet.pdf [Accessed: 2020-10-27].

[42] Zanaboni P, Wootton R. Adoption of telemedicine: from pilot stage to routine delivery. BMC Medical Informatics and Decision Making. 2012; 12:1. DOI: 10.1186/1472-6947-12-1.

[43] Greek Ministry of Health. eHealth programmes and results [Internet]. 2018. Available from: https://www.moh.gov.gr/articles/ehealth/6090-programmata-ehealth-kai-apotelesmata [Accessed: 2020-10-23].

[44] CitiesNet. United for Health [Internet]. 2015. Available from: https://dccg.gr/activites/united4health/ [Accessed: 2020-11-12].

[45] National Institution for Deaf People. Remote Interpreting Service [Internet]. 2019. Available from: https://idrimakofon.gr/relay/ [Accessed: 2020-11-10].

[46] Skai.gr. The first operation of a video-communication station for the deaf and hearing-impaired at the "Laikon" General Hospital of Attica [Internet]. 2020. Available from: https://www.skai.gr/news/technology/sto-laiko-nosokomeio-1i-leitourgia-vinteoepikoinonias-gia-kofous-kai-varikoous [Accessed: 2020-11-12].

[47] 4th Regional Health Authority Macedonia and Thrace. Press release on the launch of video-communication stations for the deaf and hearing-impaired [Internet]. 2020. Available from: https://www.4ype.gr/index.php/genika/genika/2369-stathmoi-epikoinonias-varhkoon [Accessed: 2020-11-15].

[48] World Health Organization. mHealth. New horizons through mobile technologies. Based on the findings of the second global survey on eHealth. Global Observatory for eHealth series, Volume 3 [Internet]. 2011. Available from: https://www.who.int/goe/publications/goe_mhealth_web.pdf [Accessed: 2020-11-19].

[49] European Commission. Green Paper on mobile Health ("mHealth") [Internet]. 2014. Available from: https://ec.europa.eu/digital-single-market/en/news/green-paper-mobile-health-mhealth [Accessed: 2020-10-30].

[50] McCombie A, Walmsley R, Barclay M et al. A Noninferiority Randomized Clinical Trial of the Use of the Smartphone-Based Health Applications IBDsmart and IBDoc in the Care of Inflammatory Bowel Disease Patients. Inflammatory Intestinal Diseases. 2019; 4:7-13. DOI: 10.1093/ibd/izz252.

[51] National Organization of Public Health. Psychosocial Support Hotline 10306 for the coronavirus [Internet]. 2020. Available from: https://eody.gov.gr/tilefoniki-grammi-psychokoinonikis-ypostirixis-10306-gia-ton-koronoio/ [Accessed: 2020-11-18].

[52] Kwankam SY. What e-Health can offer. Bulletin of the World Health Organization. 2004; 82:800-802.

[53] Langabeer JR, Champagne-Langabeer T, Alqusairi D et al. Cost-benefit analysis of telehealth in pre-hospital care. Journal of Telemedicine and Telecare. 2017; 23:747-751. DOI: 10.1177/1357633X16680541.

[54] Spil T, Stegwee R. Strategies for Healthcare Information Systems. In: Armoni A, editor. Effective Healthcare Information Systems. Hershey: IRM Press; 2002. pp. 1-12.

[55] European Commission. eHealth in the EU: what's the diagnosis? [Internet]. 2014. Available from: http://europa.eu/rapid/press-release_IP-14-302_en.htm [Accessed: 2021-01-04].

[56] Kallio A. eHealth and eSocial in Finland-today and 2020 [Internet]. 2015. Available from: https://ec.europa.eu/health/sites/health/files/ehealth/docs/ev_20150512_co53_en.pdf [Accessed: 2021-01-04].

[57] European Commission. State of Health in the EU. Greece. Health profile 2017 [Internet]. 2017. Available from: https://ec.europa.eu/health/sites/health/files/state/docs/chp_gr_greece.pdf [Accessed: 2020-10-19].

[58] European Commission. State of Health in the EU. Greece. Health profile

2019 [Internet]. 2019. Available from: https://ec.europa.eu/health/sites/health/files/state/docs/2019_chp_gr_greece.pdf [Accessed: 2020-10-19].

[59] Capital.gr. Rapid reduction in drug costs in the period 2009-2014 [Internet]. 2018. Available from: https://www.capital.gr/oikonomia/3272371/ragdaia-i-meiosi-stis-dapanes-gia-to-farmako-tin-periodo-2009-2014 [Accessed: 2020-11-16].

[60] European Commission. eHealth and COVID-19 [Internet]. 2020. Available from: https://ec.europa.eu/health/ehealth/covid-19_en [Accessed: 2020-11-10].

[61] Deloitte. Digital Transformation of the Health Sector [Internet]. 2020. Available from: https://www2.deloitte.com/content/dam/Deloitte/gr/Documents/life-sciences-health-care/gr_health_4_0_noexp.pdf [Accessed: 2021-01-04].

Chapter 3

Designing Disease-Specific mHealth Apps for Clinical Value

Karim Keshavjee, Dustin Johnston-Jewell, Brian Lee and Robert Kyba

Abstract

mHealth apps for patient use are promising but continue to face a plateau in usage. Current apps work for a limited segment of the patient population, i.e., those who enjoy tracking for intrinsic rewards. There are many opportunities to support patient care in between health care provider visits that are not currently being met for many diseases and patient types (personas). This is an area of great potential growth for mHealth apps and could contribute greatly to patient health and wellness. In this chapter, we propose a framework for how to think about the between-visit needs of patients that would motivate continued use of mhealth apps. We view the app design process from the following perspectives: 1) disease-specific needs, 2) non-disease specific needs, 3) behavioral theoretical aspects of app usage and 4) app-intrinsic usage motivators. Myasthenia gravis serves as the use case for illustrating these perspectives and how to use them in designing a disease-specific mHealth app.

Keywords: mHealth, user experience, design, behavior, motivation

1. Introduction

1.1 mHealth app usage remains low, in spite of increased investment

Venture investments in mobile health app development has grown 10-fold over the last 5 years, from approximately $200 million in 2014 [1] to over $2 billion in 2019 [2]. Investors are hoping to cash in on the rapidly growing mhealth app market, expected to grow at a compound annual growth rate of 21% over the next 5 years to an expected US$57 billion [3]. However, usage of mhealth apps continues to be low, especially amongst patients with chronic disease who are most likely to benefit from their use [4]. While 38% of respondents with no health condition had downloaded 1–5 mhealth apps in a recent survey, only 6.6% with hypertension had done the same. Actual usage of mhealth apps was even more abysmal, with 21% of respondents with no condition using the app 2 or more times per day compared with only 2.7% of patients with hypertension, 13% with obesity, 12.3% with diabetes and 12% with depression using the app at the same level [4]. mHealth app users are more likely to be younger and healthier with only 12% of those 55 and over using a mhealth app compared to 25% of those under 55 [5]. Interestingly, 34% of mobile users would increase their use of tracking apps if encouraged to do so by their healthcare provider (HCP) [6].

Why is app usage so low despite so much investment in the field?

1.2 There are no standards for design and development of mhealth apps

There are no standard recommendations or approaches to developing mhealth apps [7]. Several researchers and app developers have proposed design approaches, including some very generic, non-evidence-based approaches [8–10] and some based on highly respected frameworks used in other industries, such as the information systems research (ISR) framework [11, 12]. The UK government provides a thoughtful checklist of items to consider when developing an app [13].

The ISR framework recommends three cycles of iteration when designing and building an app: Relevance, Rigor and Design. Relevance speaks to what users want and need to take care of their specific health issues. Rigor implies a review of the literature to identify important information that may not have arisen during the Relevance cycle. Finally, Design speaks to user-centered design and usability evaluation. The ISR framework provides very minimal guidance around what the three cycles mean in a healthcare context. It requires starting every project using first principles, i.e., assuming nothing is known and that there are no reusable elements.

The UK government's Guide [13] to good practice for digital and data-driven technologies is a thoughtful guide to app development and includes several excellent design considerations for app publishers, including ethical considerations, defining a clear value proposition, assessing usability and accessibility, ensuring technical, clinical and data safety, regulations that should be followed, ensuring interoperability, generating evidence of impact and defining the commercialization roadmap.

These recommendations and frameworks are very generic and do not address important clinical requirements, the *raison d'etre* of mhealth app development, unless they happen to be identified during the primary research process.

All the frameworks and recommendations lack a key recommendation to improve chronic disease care: use of a behavior change theory to help drive app-related behavior change [14, 15]. They also tend to focus solely on the patient end-user and leave out a key enabler (or barrier) to app usage: the healthcare provider (HCP) [16]. The frameworks also do not specifically address the key barriers to app use [17], such as the need to 1) adapt the language and terminology used in the app to the needs of those with lower health literacy and numeracy levels. In many cases, patients with lower health literacy and numeracy do not end up participating in user engagement sessions. This can easily bias the app and leave out an important, vulnerable segment of patients who are known to use the healthcare system more often [18] and could benefit from use of the app. 2) prevent creating a large response burden on patients, i.e., asking patients to enter too much data. 3) Make the data collection and analysis relevant and actionable for the patient. 4) Make the app very easy to use so that lack of daily use does not cause loss of skill in using the app. 5) Create incentives for using the app on a regular basis; e.g., creating opportunities for social approval, cost savings, a sense of mastery or lowered anxiety. 6) Make it easy for HCPs to see that the app is scientifically valid and that it is benefitting their patients and that therefore they should encourage its use by the patient and recommend it to other patients. 7) Make it easy for HCPs to visualize the data and provide them with valuable information that saves them time during the patient encounter so that they have an incentive to recommend the app to their other patients. 8) Make it easy for the healthcare provider to incorporate the output of the app into their electronic medical record system [17].

1.3 App evaluation criteria are not design criteria

Many organizations and academics have developed criteria for evaluating apps, including the author of this paper [13, 17, 19–21]. However, no matter how comprehensive the criteria, they are both aspirational, incomplete and highly generic. For example, the very popular and highly cited Mobile Apps Rating Scale (MARS) assesses constructs such as engagement, functionality, esthetics, information and subjective quality. However, the MARS has nothing to say about disease-specific functions, integration with the healthcare system, value for healthcare providers, whether the app addresses important barriers to use or even whether the app uses behavioral theories to help with behavior change. The authors of the study even removed the concept of "evidence-based" because it was not assessed during the development of the tool. Interestingly, the authors claim that the MARS can be used as "a checklist for the design and development of new high quality health apps" [19]. The checklist is indeed useful as a general checklist of usability and user experience criteria to keep in mind when building the app but does not provide much guidance on how to design to achieve clinical benefits.

1.4 Human factors are necessary, but not sufficient for success

Most app design frameworks recommend using a human factors design approach [8–12]. These typically include 1) getting some form of input and motivations for use (user stories) from actual users and developing profiles of the different users who might use the system for a shared understanding of users (personas); some models call this the empathize step; 2) collating information from multiple sources to identify important user problems, also called the define phase in some models; 3) developing low and/or medium fidelity mock-ups and working with end users to get feedback on them; also called the ideate phase; 4) develop prototypes of the most promising ideas; called the prototype phase; 5) conducting expert usability, cognitive walkthroughs and end-user testing of the prototypes; called the test phase [22, 23].

Not surprisingly, most mhealth app developers do use human factors methods in their design process [24]. Despite using these methods, usage of mhealth apps continues to be low [4]. This is likely because human factors is only one important ingredient in a complex mix of important ingredients [17].

The International Standards Organization (ISO) has recommended a move away from user-centred design to a more human-centred design approach [25]. The name change is intended to help developers expand their focus from a single user and to start thinking more holistically about who the stakeholders of a product really are. The ISO recommends six components for human-centred design process, including: 1) documenting the needs of users and their relationships to tasks and the contexts in which they occur; 2) obtaining user involvement in all stages of design and software development; 3) obtaining on-going user feedback and conducting on-going evaluation; 4) using an iterative process for product refinement; 5) having multidisciplinary skills and diverse perspectives on the design team; and 6) ensuring the design encompasses the entire user experience (UX).

1.5 What is the role of personas in app development?

Personas have been an important part of app design for several years [26]. They enable product managers and designers to convey important information about the end-users to the development team. Personas provide product managers a structured approach to convey basic information about the different types of end-users that may use the product. What are the demographics of different users, including age, gender, geography? What are their goals, their spending habits, their needs, their pain points? What is their orientation to technology (avid, phobic or in between)? What is their attitude to the healthcare system (trusting, mistrusting, in between)? What is their relationship to their healthcare provider (want to be told what to do, want to make decisions themselves)? The persona is usually built after conducting research with users and then synthesizing a 'typical profile' of either a single ideal user or a few different types of users [27, 28].

Personas are particularly important in marketing, as they are typically built on well-researched market segments where the desired outcome (purchasing behavior) is well known [29]. Personas are essentially a mechanism to make an abstract segment more concrete for marketers, copy editors and advertising creatives. Personas have been adapted for app development, but they lack one important piece of information that is available to marketers, but not available to app developers: desired user behaviors.

Increasingly, personas are considered as caricatures and not enough for app development [30]. They are being augmented by a more powerful model popularized by Clayton Christenson: The Jobs to be Done [JTBD] framework [31, 32]. The JTBD framework posits that users do not purchase or use products for the product's sake, but rather purchase them to 'get a job done'. They 'hire' products to accomplish a task they need to complete and are looking for an outcome, rather than a feature or a function. The JTBD framework is an outcomes specification approach rather than a functional specification approach [33].

This framework provides better insight for developing functionality, because it immediately goes to the heart of why a user might want to use a product and generates a list of 'jobs to be done'. In the healthcare sector, some of the job to be done includes being able to communicate information to the HCP which the HCP considers to be relevant and easy to interpret, which is not always clear from a end-user persona perspective [34, 35].

The JTBD framework also provides guidance on identifying drivers and barriers, both rational/cognitive and affective, for using a product to get the job done [33]. This assists developers and product managers to consider unspoken barriers which inhibit the use of the product, even when the product is designed to get the 'job done'. It also assists in articulating unidentified drivers that could enhance uptake of the product but were not articulated by the end user during user-centered design sessions [33].

1.6 Apps need to follow and adapt to evidence-based guidelines for treatment and outcomes

One key reason why apps are not used is because the app makes recommendations which conflict with what HCPs communicate or believe [17]. This creates a tension for the patient: "Should I believe the app or should I believe my HCP?" Inevitably, unless the patient can find a HCP who agrees with the app, the patient realizes the app is not going to be useful, because their HCP is acting on a different set of information and therefore embarks on a different diagnostic and treatment plan than what the app recommends, rendering the app useless [36].

To make it easier for HCPs to recommend an app to patients, the HCP needs to know that the app is scientifically accurate and follows current guidelines and regulations [37]. Ideally, the app should be proven to deliver the benefits that patients desire and HCPs want to provide, however, this may be a much bigger ask than is currently possible. Our ability to evaluate apps as fast as they can change is woefully inadequate [38]. Current approaches used to evaluate drugs do not work for evaluating mhealth apps because, while drug formulations stay relatively static, mhealth apps are constantly changing.

1.7 Health behavior change is a critical component of mhealth apps

The purpose of providing patients with an mhealth app should be to improve their experiences of health care and their health outcomes [39]. If health behaviors are optimal, then adding a mhealth app may bring no additional benefit, especially if the disease has a lifestyle or behavioral component. Patients with chronic diseases which progress over time may also benefit by identifying trends earlier. mHealth apps do not have any intrinsic health properties. They, by themselves, do not lower blood pressure, treat pain or solve clinical problems. They add their value by helping patients track their relevant clinical problems, visualize their current behaviors, experiment with new behaviors and see the impact of their new behaviors on their health, including medication taking behaviors. Thus, the current short-fall in health-related behaviors (whether lifestyle or medication-related) that leads to poor health experience needs to be identified and the app needs to directly address the highest priority short-falls and those at highest risk for exhibiting poor health behaviors. It is likely that if the app is successful in addressing healthcare needs of the individual and their HCP, then the health of the user will improve, and they will no longer need the app. To maintain on-going and continuous use, app developers will need to continuously evaluate the impact of their app on patient health and add new functions to the mhealth app in future iterations.

If the app does not respond to evolving clinical needs, changes in therapy, changes in knowledge about behavior change techniques that work or changes in guidelines, the app is likely to become obsolete and lose users who increasingly experience barriers to the use of the app from their HCPs [36]. mHealth app development is a dynamic industry.

In addition to relevance and timeliness, mhealth apps need also to be built on a well-researched behavior theory. There are as many as 89 different behavior theory models that have been developed over the last several decades [15], too many to list here. However, having a theory of behavior change to underpin app features is important for several reasons: 1) you cannot change what you do not know; it's important to know current behaviors so they can be measured and tracked through the change process. 2) Understanding the mediators of behavior change allows developers to tease out whether a lack of response was due to poor design of the intervention or whether the intervention worked properly but had no impact on the relevant behavior. 3) Theories of behavior build upon a large body of knowledge and are more likely to work than a poorly informed and poorly conceptualized intervention.

Carey et al. provide a website where app developers and change agents can find links between behavior change theories and mechanisms of action [40]. Although this is an excellent service, using behavior change theories that have already been proven for a particular disease may be a much better approach than trying to pick theories based on conjecture or putative mechanisms of action [41, 42].

1.7.1 Literature review and research trump end-user engagement

Every disease is different, and every patient experiences their disease in a unique way. For example, type II diabetes is caused by a myriad of social, environmental and physiological factors related to physical activity and nutrition. In contrast, our case study disease, myasthenia gravis is an autoimmune disease that can be triggered or worsened by social, environmental and physiological factors, but is not caused by them. These differences have profound influences on what the most effective mhealth interventions are likely to be [43–48].

It is important to understand the range of behaviors that are detrimental for someone with a particular disease. Poor nutritional and exercise habits are important barriers for good health in diabetes [49], while poor medication adherence and exposure to exacerbating conditions are important considerations in myasthenia gravis, for example [50]. This type of information may be available from end-users during end-user engagement sessions, but typically requires systematic investigation by researchers and experts rather than by app developers who may miss important information because they lack expertise in a particular clinical topic [15]. Literature review and synthesis is a key requirement of mhealth app development.

1.7.2 Ability to change health behaviors requires an understanding of the range of ways that patients experience their disease

For a mhealth app to be effective, it needs to not only provide evidence-based advice, but also needs to capture and track relevant disease-specific patient behaviors. In diabetes, this is likely to be nutrition, exercise, stress, medication adherence, regular monitoring of biomarkers and sleep. In myasthenia gravis, it will include medication adherence, exposure to exacerbating factors, stress and potentially muscle strength.

Regardless of the relevant disease-specific behaviors, different patients with the same disease have different preferences and beliefs which also impact their choice of treatments, their health behaviors and approach to interacting with the healthcare system [51]. These differences in patient experience need to be considered during the app design and development process. These differences can be captured as part of the persona development process.

1.8 App-related behavior change is not health behavior change

How users relate to apps is very different from the way they relate to their disease. Health-related behaviors are highly dependent on the nature of the disease, while app related behaviors are dependent on characteristics of the app and the clinical setting; i.e., ease of use, user experience, getting the job done and a sense of accountability to the HCP and the healthcare team.

A significant majority of mhealth apps do not use a theoretical basis for driving behavior change [52]. Geuens et al. [53] describe a tool which links behavior change theories to mhealth app features to make it easer for developers to incorporate behavior change theories into their applications [54]. The features in the Trustworthiness and Liking section are all related to better app use. An excellent and comprehensive list of methods to improve app usability mentions many good techniques to improve app usability and the user experience, including 1) minimizing cognitive load, 2) minimizing response burden, 3) breaking down tasks into smaller sub-tasks, 4) making it easy to navigate and know where you are in the app, etc. [55].

1.9 Not all patients are alike. Patient segmentation is necessary for personalizing care

Not all patient segmentation approaches are relevant to mhealth app design. For example, the approach recommended by Brommels [56] which breaks down patients into 7 categories (healthy, incidental, chronic disease, multi-morbid, needing elective treatment, trauma, requiring hospitalization) is more suited to health delivery systems and how to segment patients for health delivery planning. The approach used by Deloitte who categorize health consumers into 4 categories (trailblazers, prospectors, bystanders and homesteaders) is more suited to understanding patients as consumers and purchasers of healthcare as opposed to as individuals who are purchasing a product to solve a problem [57].

What app developers need is a method to segment patients to enable more personalized solutions and communications for patients [51]. A Finnish organization has developed such a segmentation approach for Diabetes [58] and Sandy et al. developed one for hypertension [59]. Ideally, app developers should find a well-researched patient segmentation approach for the disease for which they are building an app.

1.10 Ecological momentary assessments and interventions are useful theoretical constructs

There's a lot of hype about using sensors embedded in smartphones to detect changes in usage patterns which imply a worsening of disease [60] or for detection of disease [61–63]. Even very recent studies are exploratory and need additional validation before being translated into the field [64, 65]. Although the research base that makes production use of smartphone sensors is still in its infancy [66], there are some promising developments in creating architectures that are ready for conducting research. Digital (behavior) phenotyping, the ability to use wearables and sensor data to detect different behaviors, is developing rapidly and it is likely that the basic science will become more easily accessible over the next several years [67]. The developers of the geographically explicit ecological momentary assessment (GEMA) architecture claim that their approach is scalable from their study in post-partum mothers to other disease areas [68].

The use of validated patient reported measures questionnaires for conducting ecological momentary assessments is well developed and can be used with good design in terms of frequency and response burden [69, 70]. Patient reported experience and outcomes measures (PREMS and PROMS) have been developed in a variety of disease areas and are a promising way for mhealth app developers to get a jump start on ecological momentary assessments [71–74]. Use of PREMS and PROMS may incur a license fee but are worth the cost since the tools are generally validated and are widely used in clinical trials. Care must be taken to select PREMS and PROMs properly, since some of them are more useful as aggregate measures (suitable for clinical trials) but are not appropriate for use on individual patients in a clinical setting [75].

Ecological momentary interventions are another promising concept, especially in the mental health field, where cognitive and affective interventions can be delivered directly through an app [76–78]. Although it is possible for apps to be used for other interventions, such as driving insulin pumps in response to readings from a continuous glucose monitoring system [79] this is still unusual and very much in its infancy.

Ecological momentary interventions are also very promising for delivering behavior change interventions at just the right time [80]. Ideally, delivery of interventions should be timed to when people are most receptive to receiving them. Timing of interventions can be predicted by use of ecological momentary assessments to know when a patient might be at their worst or at their best and deliver an intervention at just the right time [81, 82].

1.11 Effectiveness assessment requires a rapid research infrastructure and new research methodologies

Many app guidelines request app developers to test their app for clinical benefits [13, 83]. However, testing apps can be a fraught process, because typically, apps are designed and developed using an agile process, but clinical evaluation requires a more waterfall process. The methodologies for development and evaluation are somewhat incompatible and creates friction for good quality clinical trials. Philpott et al. make some recommendations about how to create a clinical trials infrastructure that is more flexible to the needs of mobile health app evaluation. They recommend a 2-phase approach. The first phase is a qualitative phase with usability and expert reviews to ensure that the app meets minimum criteria for more rigorous testing. The second phase then evaluates the app in an adaptive randomized controlled trial, which allows low quality apps to be identified and quickly removed from the study and allows high quality apps to be tested more rigorously [38]. This ensures that scarce resources are not wasted on apps that do not add value.

2. Use case: myasthenia gravis

Myasthenia gravis (MG) is a chronic autoimmune disease that targets the neuromuscular junction and causes unpredictable, fluctuating muscle weakness. Symptoms include drooping eyelids (the classical, textbook symptom), difficulty breathing, upper and lower limb weakness, difficulty swallowing and slurred speech [84]. MG affects about 20 people in every 100,000 [85]. It is twice more prevalent in women who get it in their 20s–30s than in men who get it in their 60s–80s. At one time, the mortality rate for MG was as high as 75%. However, with advances in treatment, the mortality rate is down to less than 5% [85]. Patients with MG are treated by neurologists.

We use myasthenia gravis as the use case for demonstrating a framework for designing the clinical aspects of a mobile health app.

2.1 Identifying and designing for disease-specific needs

Patient focus groups were formed before any app development activities were started to get patient input on whether an app would add value and if so, what the app should encompass. Patients agreed that an app could fill a gap that exists in care. They provided information about their experience of their disease and provided high level guidance about the features, functionality and benefits they would like to see in an app.

Clinician (neurologist) key informant interviews (N=8) were held to gather clinician experiences and gather clinician input into what they would like to see in an app for MG. Clinicians indicated that they struggle with capturing important information about the patient's disease progression, medication use and compliance and the broad range of quality-of-life issues that patients with MG face. Clinicians are also interested in learning more about objective physical signs and not just the subjective patient experience. Key clinician-anticipated benefits from an app include getting a better, more detailed timeline of key events without the fog of recall bias and getting a better sense of medication compliance. There was no consensus on how to track patients between visits, but everyone knew about the MG Activities of Daily Living questionnaire (MG-ADL) [86]. Clinicians indicated that an app would also benefit primary care physicians, who are taking on more of the care of patients with MG.

Key neurology opinion leaders (N=7) were also interviewed to better understand the context in which the app would be introduced, what metrics the app would need to exhibit for them to support it and reasons they would need to recommend it to other clinicians.

2.1.1 Experiences of patients with MG

Patients with MG have unique disease-specific experiences. They experience anxiety (from the uncertainty of their disease) and social negativity (forced withdrawal from normal social activities). They experience stigma, deconditioning and exhaustion. Many experience stigmatizing side-effects of the medication, such as obesity, skin rashes and poor mood. Many experience disability and are unable to work.

There are 3 possible reasons that patients experience worsening of symptoms: 1) a worsening of the underlying disease process leading to worsening of symptoms, 2) poor compliance to medication and 3) patient is experiencing exacerbating factors, such as stress, lack of sleep, extreme heat or cold, contraindicated medications and viral illness.

Although one benefit of using an app could be that patients receive an escalation in treatment sooner, many patients paradoxically fear dose escalation because of the side effects they experience from using some medications. It is hoped that better tracking of exacerbating factors could help minimize dose escalations by identifying triggers for worsening of symptoms, other than a worsening of disease. All these assertions would, of course, need to be tested.

We combined disease-specific factors and patient motivations to create 4 personas: 1) The In-Charge is a user with intrinsic motivation to use the app because they like to collect data and analyze it for insights that they can act upon themselves. 2) The Worrier is anxious about the disease, the symptoms they experience, how the medication makes them feel, how they will cope if things get worse and the uncertainty of when the next exacerbation will occur. They also worry about how others perceive them and the loss of control they have over their lives because of MG. 3) The Adaptive Manager seeks to control events by gathering as much information as possible and partnering with their doctor to be proactive and manage their disease in the best way possible. And 4) the Passive Monitor who collects information because their doctor has asked them to do so. They trust that if their doctor thinks it is a good thing, then it must be so. There is of course a fifth persona: The Non-User. The Non-User does not believe that an app can be of enough benefit to make it worth their while to use.

2.1.2 App design considerations

The key underlying premise for developing the MG mhealth app was to help patients track their symptoms, treatments and exacerbating factors in between visits to their doctor so that they can self-manage their disease better and so that their HCP can review information in the app to get a more accurate and more comprehensive summary of what happened since their last visit. We selected the validated MG quality of life tool called the Myasthenia Gravis Activities of Daily Living profile (MG-ADL) [86] to capture data about patient symptoms. The app also allows tracking of some common physical activities such as walking the dog or climbing stairs which are important to the patient. This provides them with the ability to track how well they are doing for important activities which may not be considered to be 'activities of daily living'.

Benefits and goals of tracking symptoms, medication use, health system use and exacerbating factors we identified included, 1) patients may identify reasons for disease worsening earlier with use of the app and, in some cases, be able to act on the information themselves; e.g., get more sleep or avoid situations which make their disease worse (benefit to In-Charge and Adaptive Manager). 2) Patients may make the visit with their HCP more efficient and productive, giving them more time to ask questions that are important to them (benefits Worrier, Adaptive Manager). 3) Patients may receive treatment escalation sooner, if the HCP is better able to tease out worsening of underlying disease from a string of bad days (benefits all patient types). These benefits are communicated to the patient throughout the app, to remind them of the benefits and reinforce use of the app.

Most patients (75% of women and 56% of men) do not like the side-effects of prednisone and resist dose escalations [87]. Making it easy for patients to capture more granular information about their medication use may be helpful for physicians to tailor doses and minimize the dose escalations or minimize the duration of a dose escalation. Rather than asking patients to enter all their medication data into the app and track detailed usage, it may be as valuable to capture the main 2 most problematic medications used in the treatment of MG and ask the patient periodically whether they used it as prescribed and if not, why not. That information would be easier for the patient to enter and may be just as helpful to the HCP as a much more detailed log of medication use.

Fear, uncertainty, change and stigma are a big part of the MG experience [88]. Using more reassuring and calming language, without promising anything that cannot be delivered by the app is a good way of addressing anxiety. A root cause of stigma is ignorance. Providing useful facts about MG to the patient about self-management and how to explain their disease to others could help decrease uncertainty and stigma and help the patient cope better with unavoidable change. These facts and messages can be entered into a fact and message bank that can be displayed to the patient randomly, helping to keep the app fresh and educating patients at the same time. In future iterations, the app may wish to include an optional cognitive behavioral therapy component and/or a mood or anxiety tracker.

Patients who desire more control over the app (In-Charge and Adaptive Manager) are given an opportunity to make changes to the settings for a variety of features. Expert review identified that some of the features that patients could control (for example, what would be released to their HCP in the report) would only increase their anxiety and have a paradoxical effect on patients perceived control over the app. It was recommended that the control over the HCP report be removed as it did not impact the patient. The reports provided to patients were also harmonized to look more like what was provided to the physician so that they would not be disoriented when having a conversation with their HCP.

Patients with MG frequently experience exhaustion, which is independent of muscle weakness, the hallmark of the disease. This means that patients with MG spend a lot of time in bed, unable to move, but still able to think and perform cognitive tasks. We recommended that the app provide a function to lock the aspect ratio so that patients can view the app in the more convenient portrait mode while lying down.

Almost half of patients with MG experience reduced social positivity and physical activity, increasing their chances of becoming depressed and becoming deconditioned. Future iterations of the app will consider adding a gratitude journal and/or a cognitive behavioral therapy component. Future iterations could also provide the patient with a physical activity program to prevent physical deconditioning.

2.2 Identifying and designing for non-disease-specific drivers and barriers

Patients experience many frictions to use of apps [17]. A small segment of approximately 20% of the app-using population has an intrinsic motivation to use an app [89]. They track their disease on a regular basis from an internal motivation with little encouragement – they will use an app if you offer them one. Another 34% of users say they would use an app if their doctor recommended it [6]. Making the app useful to HCP will make it more likely that HCP will endorse and encourage use. We addressed the following issues in our design.

2.2.1 App provides information that conflicts with information received from HCP

We designed the app to be consistent with current guidelines or current standards of practice in MG. Unfortunately, the current MG treatment guidelines are not well-respected and utilized. In this case, we asked our clinical advisors to provide us with the latest information about diagnosis, treatment and management of patients with MG. The clinical advisors provided guidance to include simple medication and health system outcome tracking which is important to doctors. It will be important to ensure that app maintenance includes regular check-ins with neurologists to update the app to current standards of practice.

2.2.2 Language and terminology of the app not compatible with the patient's health literacy

We simplified the language used in the app. Although it is very difficult to translate all medical issues to a grade 6 level, where possible, we minimized use of difficult words and used the same difficult terminology in different contexts so that users would learn their meanings after repeated use. We repeated important concepts to reinforce learning. We used language that was compatible with the 4 different personas we identified (see below). We also reframed messages on goals and outcomes to appeal to the various types of users.

2.2.3 Patient must enter the data himself or herself

We minimized data entry tasks and burden (aka response burden) by asking patients to identify what was important to them. Although the questionnaire is relatively short at only 8-questions, not all questions are relevant to all patients. In a clinical trial setting, there is no option but to use the entire scale because missing data can easily invalidate a study. However, for an app that tracks the individual effectiveness of clinical treatment, focusing on what's most important to the patient can go a long way to decreasing response burden and increasing compliance to data capture; some data is always better than no data. The purpose of the app is not to capture data, but to help the patient manage their disease and to track the trajectory of their disease. If the patient rarely or never experiences a particular symptom, there is no need to track that information. If patients experience their worst symptoms in a particular part of their body, then tracking that symptom may be an excellent sentinel event for tracking overall disease state. Using this approach, we were able to decrease the number of questions that the patient had to answer.

Another way to reduce response burden is to ask patients to fill out the questionnaire randomly spread out over a longer period. By 'sampling' the patient's disease experience over a longer period, it is possible to get a good sense of the patient's disease trajectory and then sample more or less frequently to optimize the amount of information compared to the response burden for the patient.

The magnitude and/or the magnitude of change in patient responses can also be used to make data entry more meaningful to the patient. If the patient's symptoms are low and/or stable, the app can take longer to notify the patient to enter data. If the patient's symptoms are worse or changing, then capturing data more frequently makes more sense and is likely to be more acceptable to the patient.

2.2.4 Patient cannot use information in a meaningful way

Patients generally have little control over their clinical condition. They cannot order diagnostic testing, prescribe medications or refer themselves to specialists. They are dependent to a great extent on their HCPs for those clinical actions. However, it does not mean that they have no control over their condition.

In myasthenia gravis, the patient has 1 major concern on a day-to-day basis: when my symptoms worsen on any one day, am I just having a 'bad day' or is it a worsening of my underlying condition? The uncertainty of symptom worsening can be a great source of anxiety [88]. The app could help patients see the trends of their disease and help them better and more quickly distinguish between a 'bad day' and a worsening of their disease, thereby giving them greater control over their disease experience.

The other way that patients can be empowered to use the app is to provide an easy-to-use report from the app for their HCP. This report, if useful and used by the HCP, would benefit the patient directly. Because of the uncertainty and daily variation in symptoms experienced by patients with MG, recalling their symptoms and experience of their disease during a visit with their HCP can be challenging. This was confirmed by our panel of clinical experts who indicated that history taking in MG is challenging and time-consuming. HCPs are likely to benefit from and value a simple, easy to read, visual report of the patient's symptoms overlaid with information about compliance to medication and exacerbating factors experienced at the time of symptom worsening. Since, this is the most beneficial information for HCP, we need only capture medication compliance and exacerbating factor information at the time of symptom worsening, thereby minimizing response burden further.

Patients are influenced by non-verbal cues from their HCP. If the HCP does not use the information in the report, they are likely to stop using the app. However, if patients perceive that HCPs value the reports, they will continue using the app. HCPs have a strong influence on patient app usage and can reinforce app usage by requesting the report and by viewing the information and acting on in it, where appropriate.

2.2.5 Lack of incentives like cost saving or social approval

There are few external incentives for using an app in MG. MG is not a lifestyle disease, so getting empathy from other people is rather difficult. MG is also a stigmatizing disease (see below), so social sharing of progress may not be appropriate or desired by the patient. However, there is a useful behavior change theory called the Self-determination Theory (SDT) [90] which was determined to be appropriate for patients with MG and could provide a significant incentive to use the app. How SDT was incorporated into the app is described below in Section 2.3.

2.2.6 Daily use of the app is not required and therefore patient does not get into the habit of using it

Although patients with MG can experience symptoms at any time, the lived reality is that exacerbations and improvements play out over weeks and months.

Collecting data everyday can become tedious and lead to response fatigue. How do we design an app that maintains a good balance between infrequent data collection and loss of skill over time?

Through Expert Usability reviews, we simplified the data collection so that patients only reported data about the symptoms that are most troublesome to them. We also simplified the task loops so that they could get feedback from their data entry in smaller cycles of data entry, instead of getting one big report after answering a long series of questions. Encouraging and educational messages are spread throughout the data entry tasks so that patients do not get fatigued with answering many questions. Messages that explain the rationale for capturing specific information can help the patient connect the data they are entering to the outcomes they are hoping to achieve.

Notifications can help remind the patient to track information. To improve response rates, the notification could be developed to enable data entry directly into the notification rather than having to open the app and enter the data there. This is particularly useful where a single response is required, such as 'Did you take your medications as prescribed yesterday?' It is better to ask a question like that about a completed time unit rather than asking it for an incomplete time unit, since there is a finite chance that the patient may not have completed a task that the app is asking about.

2.2.7 HCPs may not value or use the data collected by patients in apps whose provenance and pedigree is not known or established

It is important that HCPs understand how the app was designed, who was involved in the design and what evidence was used to guide its development. More importantly, this information will be more credible and trustworthy if they hear it from their peers and key opinion leaders they look to for knowledge about new products in their field. If HCPs are convinced about the benefits of the app for themselves and their patients, based on reports from opinion leaders who have already tested the app in their own practices, the more likely it is that they will be the ones to recommend it to patients in the first place, obviating this barrier.

2.2.8 There is no way for HCPs to consume the large amounts of data that are collected in apps

HCPs do not have time to download data from an app, clean it up, analyze it and visualize it during a patient encounter. The entire task needs to be done for them before the patient even arrives at the clinic. It should already be in the patient's electronic medical record when the HCP is reviewing the chart. The app should generate a simple report that the patient can email to their HCP so it can be attached to the record by the time the patient arrives.

The report should summarize the data from the previous 3–6 months since the last visit and should provide the HCP with actionable information. Do the exacerbations point to a worsening of disease or just poor control on the part of the patient? Is the poor control because of poor compliance to medication or due to exacerbating factors? If the HCP can answer these two main questions, they can have a more fruitful discussion about the patient's goals and how they can be achieved, rather than spending most of their time sorting out what happened since the last visit.

2.2.9 HCP is unable to integrate app data into their own EMR for analysis or follow-up or share the data in their EMR with their patient's apps

The current state of interoperability in most jurisdictions has not matured to the point where this type of digital data exchange can occur easily or quickly. HL7's Fast

Healthcare Interoperability Resources (FHIR) standard is evolving rapidly and is likely to be readily available over the next 5–10 years. As of late 2021, it is relatively immature and not ready for production use with apps.

2.3 Identifying and designing for a behavior-theoretical model

Through a process of discussion, reflection and mapping the experience of patients with MG to various behavior change theories, we determined the Self-determination Theory (SDT) [90] to be appropriate for patients with MG. SDT posits that people have a need for personal growth and that there are 3 intrinsic motivators that drive that growth: 1) A need for mastery over life's situations (Competence); 2) a need to feel in control over our lives (Autonomy); and 3) a need to feel connected to others (Relatedness).

SDT has a strong connection to the lived experiences of people with MG. Many patients with MG want to have more control over their lives and be able to do that through more knowledge and skills about their disease. They also want to gain greater connectedness to their HCP to get better guidance on how to manage their disease and faster time to treatment. The incentive for using the app should be rooted in a behavior theory that is compatible with improvement of the disease experience.

We incorporated the 3 elements of the SDT by providing more facts and information that the patient can use to manage their disease, by providing visualizations of the data they collect to help them see how well they are doing and what they can do to improve their disease experience and providing them with a concise and easy to understand report suitable for sharing with their HCP, thereby promoting control and relatedness at the same time. These factors can be refined over time, as patients start interacting with the app in the real-world.

2.4 Identifying and designing for app-related behaviors

App-related behaviors were considered at various stages of app use: 1) during on-boarding, 2) when capturing baseline data, 3) during routine use. The Elaboration Likelihood Model and the Information-Motivation Behavioral Skills model are excellent behavior change models for use in mhealth app design and development as the focus on app-related behaviors [54].

The Elaboration Likelihood Model (ELM) states that behavior change will usually arise after a change in one's beliefs and attitudes and that a change in beliefs and attitudes can be triggered by a cognitive stimulus, i.e., a message or fact. The ELM proposes several mechanisms for delivering the cognitive stimulus, including *personalization*, *verifiability*, *expertise* and *surface credibility*.

The Information-Motivation Behavioral Skills (IMB) model states that new behaviors are the result of information, motivation and skill in executing a behavior. The IMB proposes the following mechanisms for delivering relevant information, motivations and skills to patients: *reduction* of effort needed to do something, *tunneling* to breakdown large goals into smaller, more manageable goals, *reminders* that help the patient remember to do a task and *macro tailoring* which means adapting messages to the needs of a specific group or segment.

During on-boarding, we want to make it fun and easy for users to start using the app. The first few screens do not require any data entry (*reduction*). They inform the patient about the app, explain the benefits of using the app from the perspective of all the different personas (*macro tailoring*) and start educating the patient about how to use the app and what to expect from using the app. The app's design is very professional and has a clean and visually appealing look and feel, giving the app *surface credibility*. The patient also learns that the app has been developed by experts in the field (*expertise*).

When capturing baseline data, the patient is offered some control over what they would like to track and share with their HCP (*personalization*). Although all patients are asked to enter the minimum data that will generate a report for the HCP, they have the option of only capturing relevant information about their symptoms. Once they have entered a small amount of data, they are offered a visualization of their information (*tunneling*). Baseline capture occurs on the first day of use. The aim is to keep the session relatively short and pleasant, even though the patient is likely to be excited about using the app for the first time and would be willing to spend a lot more time with the app. Allowing the patient to get too excited could lead to overinflated expectations and disappointment.

Once the patient has entered their baseline information, they enter the routine use phase. During this phase, they can explore the app, learn about their disease and learn about the provenance of the information made available to them (*verifiability*). They also receive notifications to enter data periodically (*reminders*) and can change the settings to personalize the schedule of notifications.

3. Conclusion

This chapter contributes new knowledge about how to design the clinical components of a mobile health app. It does not replace existing guidelines and frameworks for mobile app development in general and mhealth apps specifically. Rather, it complements existing approaches and adds new information that may be helpful for app developers when designing the disease-specific features and functions of an mHealth app. Specifically, it adds the following to our current knowledge about designing mhealth apps: 1) It makes a distinction between disease-specific behaviors and needs and non-disease-specific barriers and needs. This enables app designers to dig down deeper into specific health-related experiences and encourages them to identify information in the literature which might illuminate app development. It provides a list of common barriers to mhealth app use and potential solutions to those barriers. 2) It makes a distinction between disease-related behaviors and app related behaviors. These are two very different types of behaviors and should have different design approaches, including use of different behavior change theories to underpin them.

This chapter also brings together several existing concepts and design patterns into a more coherent mhealth app design approach. We identify that human factors methodology is necessary but not sufficient for app development and recommend the expansion of user-centred design to human-centred design that considers a wider group of stakeholders, especially the HCP and the opinion leaders who influence them. We complement the use of personas with the Jobs to be Done framework and explain the key limitation of using personas in the design of apps compared to their use in marketing. We elaborate on the use of patient segmentation using disease-specific criteria, rather than generic or health-system level segmentation as a way of meeting the needs of different patient types and different app user types.

The limitations of this framework include the fact that the outcomes of using the framework have not been tested in the real-world and that there are two issues that the framework does not address. These include no research-based or proven guidance on 1) how to make a mhealth app engaging or 2) how to make an app visually appealing. In addition, we did not include any guidance on behavioral economic theory and choice architecture, also known as 'nudge theory' [91].

Overall, we believe this chapter will help app developers and publishers to build better apps that consider the disease-specific needs of patients and use behavior theories more effectively by conceptualizing disease-specific behaviors and app-specific behaviors as qualitatively different and therefore making apps more useful to patients and their caregivers.

Acknowledgements

We would like to thank Patrick Glinski at Normative for his support in the development of the app.

Conflict of interest

Karim Keshavjee was a consultant on the project to develop the app. Dustin Johnston-Jewell and Brian Lee work at Normative.

Author details

Karim Keshavjee[1*], Dustin Johnston-Jewell[2], Brian Lee[2] and Robert Kyba[3]

1 University of Toronto, InfoClin Inc., Toronto, ON, Canada

2 Normative Inc., Toronto, ON, Canada

3 Strategic Global Counsel Inc., Toronto, ON, Canada

*Address all correspondence to: karim.keshavjee@utoronto.ca

References

[1] Pai, A., 2021. Mobile Health Investors [online] MobiHealthNews. Available at: shorturl.at/sNW28 [Accessed 5 April 2021].

[2] Mercom Capital Group, 2021. mHealth Companies Raised $2.2 Billion in Venture Funding in 2019 – Mercom Capital Group [online] Mercom Capital Group. Available at: shorturl.at/eDMN3 [Accessed 5 April 2021].

[3] Fortune Insights, 2021. mHealth apps market size is projected to reach USD 57.57 billion [online] GlobeNewswire news room. Available at: Shorturl.at/lzAL0 [Accessed 5 April 2021].

[4] Robbins R, Krebs P, Jagannathan R, Jean-Louis G, Duncan DT. Health app use among US Mobile phone users: Analysis of trends by chronic disease status. JMIR mhealth Uhealth 2017;5(12):e197. URL: https://mhealth.jmir.org/2017/12/e197 DOI:10.2196/mhealth.7832

[5] McCarthy, J., 2019. One in five U.S. adults use health apps, wearable trackers [online] Gallup.com. Available at: <shorturl.at/ptxB8> [Accessed 13 April 2021].

[6] Rupp, S., 2021. Mobiquity study: 70 percent of people track their health and fitness daily with Mobile apps – Electronic health reporter [online] Electronichealthreporter.com. Available at: <tinyurl.com/n748db4> [Accessed 10 May 2021].

[7] Adu MD, Malabu UH, Callander EJ, Malau-Aduli AE, Malau-Aduli BS. Considerations for the Development of Mobile Phone Apps to Support Diabetes Self-Management: Systematic Review. JMIR Mhealth Uhealth. 2018 Jun 21;6(6):e10115. DOI:10.2196/10115. PMID: 29929949; PMCID: PMC6035345

[8] Tuan, J., 2021. 6 Best Practices To Improve Your Mobile Health App | Healthcare IT Today [online] Healthcare IT Today | Fresh, Daily, Practical Healthcare IT Insights. Available at: <shorturl.at/inyP7> [Accessed 6 April 2021].

[9] Wicklund, E., 2021. How to Design and Develop a Mobile Health Application [online] mHealthIntelligence. Available at: <shorturl.at/wJW37> [Accessed 13 April 2021].

[10] Kays Harbor Technologies. 2016. Designing healthcare apps: 10 best practices to follow | Kays Harbor [online] Available at: <shorturl.at/kuyWX> [Accessed 13 April 2021].

[11] Farao J, Malila B, Conrad N, Mutsvangwa T, Rangaka MX, Douglas TS. A user-centred design framework for mHealth. PLoS One. 2020 Aug 19;15(8):e0237910. DOI:10.1371/journal.pone.0237910.

[12] Carballo-Dieguez A, Carry M, Gelaude D, Mosley JP, Travers J. A user-centered model for designing consumer mobile health (mHealth) applications (apps). J Biomed Inform. 2016 Apr;60:243-251. DOI:10.1016/j.jbi.2016.02.002. Epub 2016 Feb 20.

[13] GOV.UK. 2021. A guide to good practice for digital and data-driven health technologies [online] Available at: <https://tinyurl.com/abmsrjjv> [Accessed 8 May 2021].

[14] Swann C, Rosenbaum S, Lawrence A, Vella SA, McEwan D, Ekkekakis P. Updating goal-setting theory in physical activity promotion: A critical conceptual review. Health Psychol Rev. 2021 Mar;15(1):34-50. DOI:10.1080/17437199.2019.1706616. Epub 2020 Jan 27. PMID: 31900043.

[15] Davis R, Campbell R, Hildon Z, Hobbs L, Michie S. Theories of

behaviour and behaviour change across the social and behavioural sciences: a scoping review. Health Psychol Rev. 2015;9(3):323-44. DOI:10.1080/17437199.2014.941722. Epub 2014 Aug 8. PMID: 25104107; PMCID: PMC4566873.

[16] Rees S, Williams A. Promoting and supporting self-management for adults living in the community with physical chronic illness: A systematic review of the effectiveness and meaningfulness of the patient-practitioner encounter. JBI Libr Syst Rev. 2009;7(13):492-582. DOI:10.11124/01938924-200907130-00001. PMID: 27819974.

[17] Chindalo P, Karim A, Brahmbhatt R, Saha N, Keshavjee K. Health apps by design: A reference architecture for mobile engagement. InHealth care delivery and clinical science: Concepts, methodologies, tools, and applications 2018 (pp. 553-563). IGI Global.

[18] Fiscella K, Williams DR. Health disparities based on socioeconomic inequities: Implications for urban health care. Acad Med. 2004 Dec;79(12):1139-1147. DOI:10.1097/00001888-200412000-00004. PMID: 15563647.

[19] Stoyanov SR, Hides L, Kavanagh DJ, Zelenko O, Tjondronegoro D, Mani M Mobile App Rating Scale: A new tool for assessing the quality of health Mobile apps. JMIR Mhealth Uhealth 2015;3(1):e27. DOI:10.2196/mhealth.3422

[20] Hensher M, Cooper P, Dona SWA, Angeles MR, Nguyen D, Heynsbergh N, Chatterton ML, Peeters A. Scoping review: Development and assessment of evaluation frameworks of mobile health apps for recommendations to consumers. J Am Med Inform Assoc. 2021 Mar 31:ocab041. DOI:10.1093/jamia/ocab041. Epub ahead of print. PMID: 33787894.

[21] Lagan S, Sandler L, Torous J. Evaluating evaluation frameworks: a scoping review of frameworks for assessing health apps. BMJ Open. 2021 Mar 19;11(3):e047001. DOI:10.1136/bmjopen-2020-047001. PMID: 33741674; PMCID: PMC7986656.

[22] Harte R, Glynn L, Rodríguez-Molinero A, Baker PM, Scharf T, Quinlan LR, ÓLaighin G. A human-Centered design methodology to enhance the usability, human factors, and user experience of connected health systems: A three-phase methodology. JMIR Hum Factors 2017;4(1):e8 DOI:10.2196/humanfactors.5443

[23] Doorley, S., Holcomb, S., Klebahn, P., Segovia, K. and Utley, J., 2021. Design thinking bootleg — Stanford d.school [online] Stanford d.school. Available at: <https://dschool.stanford.edu/resources/design-thinking-bootleg> [Accessed 11 May 2021].

[24] Baysari MT, Westbrook JI. Mobile Applications for Patient-centered Care Coordination: A Review of Human Factors Methods Applied to their Design, Development, and Evaluation. Yearb Med Inform. 2015 Aug 13;10(1):47-54. DOI:10.15265/IY-2015-011. PMID: 26293851; PMCID: PMC4587034.

[25] International Organization for Standardization. 2017. ISO 9241--210:2010. https://www.iso.org/standard/52075.html (2017)

[26] Olsen, M., 2004. Making Personas More Powerful: Details to Drive Strategic and Tactical Design – Boxes and Arrows [online] Boxes and Arrows. Available at: <https://tinyurl.com/2wwkzkvt> [Accessed 13 May 2021].

[27] Lau, K., 2018. Personas and User Journeys in Health [online] Medium. Available at: <https://uxplanet.org/personas-and-user-journeys-in-health-b4f4596f428d> [Accessed 13 May 2021].

[28] Neate T, Bourazeri A, Roper A, Stumpf S, Wilson S. Co-created personas: Engaging and empowering users with diverse needs within the design process. InProceedings of the 2019 CHI conference on human factors in computing systems 2019 May 2 (pp. 1-12).

[29] France, H., 2020. How To Create Personas For Marketing In 2021 | Digital Agency Network [online] Digital Agency Network. Available at: <https://tinyurl.com/29xf5r9w> [Accessed 13 May 2021].

[30] McKeen, J., 2019. The pitfalls of personas and advantages of jobs to Be done: UXmatters [online] Uxmatters.com. Available at: <https://tinyurl.com/4z6nhaff> [Accessed 10 May 2021].

[31] Christensen, C., Hall, T., Dillon, K. and Duncan, D., 2016. Know Your Customers' "Jobs to Be Done" [online] Harvard Business Review. Available at: <https://tinyurl.com/32ebycxm> [Accessed 10 May 2021].

[32] Abraham, M., 2016. My product management toolkit (10): jobs-to-be-done [online] Medium. Available at: <https://tinyurl.com/2brbnv7r> [Accessed 10 May 2021].

[33] Ulwick, T., 2021. Jobs-to-be-Done: A Framework for Customer Needs [online] Medium. Available at: <https://tinyurl.com/56bwwwwj> [Accessed 10 May 2021].

[34] Sedlmayr B, Schöffler J, Prokosch HU, Sedlmayr M. User-centered design of a mobile medication management. Inform Health Soc Care. 2019;44(2):152-163. DOI:10.1080/17538157.2018.1437042. Epub 2018 Mar 5. PMID: 29504838.

[35] Amann J, Fiordelli M, Brach M, Bertschy S, Scheel-Sailer A, Rubinelli S. Co-designing a Self-Management App Prototype to Support People With Spinal Cord Injury in the Prevention of Pressure Injuries: Mixed Methods Study. JMIR Mhealth Uhealth. 2020 Jul 9;8(7):e18018. DOI:10.2196/18018. PMID: 32673241; PMCID: PMC7380902.

[36] Bierbrier, R., Lo, V., & Wu, R. C. (2014). Evaluation of the accuracy of smartphone medical calculation apps. Journal of Medical Internet Research, 16(2), e32. doi:10.2196/jmir.3062 PMID:24491911

[37] Fleming GA, Petrie JR, Bergenstal RM, Holl RW, Peters AL, Heinemann L. Diabetes digital app technology: Benefits, challenges, and recommendations. A consensus report by the European Association for the Study of diabetes (EASD) and the American Diabetes Association (ADA) diabetes technology working group. Diabetologia. 2020 Feb;63(2):229-241. DOI:10.1007/s00125-019-05034-1. PMID: 31802144.

[38] Philpott D, Guergachi A, Keshavjee K. Design and validation of a platform to evaluate mHealth apps. Stud Health Technol Inform. 2017;235:3-7. PMID: 28423744.

[39] Obucina M, Harris N, Fitzgerald JA, Chai A, Radford K, Ross A, Carr L, Vecchio N. The application of triple aim framework in the context of primary healthcare: A systematic literature review. Health Policy. 2018 Aug;122(8):900-907. DOI:10.1016/j.healthpol.2018.06.006. Epub 2018 Jun 18. PMID: 29935730.

[40] Carey RN, Connell Bohlen L, Johnston M, Rothman A, de Bruin M, Kelly MP, et al. Behaviour change techniques and their mechanisms of action: a synthesis of links described in published intervention literature 2018. doi:10.1093/abm/kay078. Available at <https://theoryandtechniquetool.humanbehaviourchange.org/.> [Accessed 10 May 2021].

[41] Kwan YH, Cheng TY, Yoon S, Ho LYC, Huang CW, Chew EH, Thumboo J, Østbye T, Low LL. A systematic review of nudge theories and strategies used to influence adult health behaviour and outcome in diabetes management. Diabetes Metab. 2020 Nov;46(6):450-460. DOI:10.1016/j.diabet.2020.04.002. Epub 2020 May 6. PMID: 32387700.

[42] Sittig S, McGowan A, Iyengar S. Extensive review of persuasive system design categories and principles: Behavioral obesity interventions. J Med Syst. 2020 Jun 5;44(7):128. DOI:10.1007/s10916-020-01591-w. PMID: 32500161.

[43] Wali S, Keshavjee K, Nguyen L, Mbuagbaw L, Demers C. Using an Electronic App to Promote Home-Based Self-Care in Older Patients With Heart Failure: Qualitative Study on Patient and Informal Caregiver Challenges. JMIR Cardio. 2020 Nov 9;4(1):e15885. DOI:10.2196/15885. Erratum in: JMIR Cardio. 2020 Nov 11;4(1):e25624. PMID: 33164901; PMCID: PMC7657601.

[44] Tassone C, Keshavjee K, Paglialonga A, Moreira N, Pinto J, Quintana Y. Evaluation of mobile apps for treatment of patients at risk of developing gestational diabetes. Health Informatics J. 2020 Sep;26(3):1983-1994. DOI:10.1177/1460458219896639. Epub 2020 Jan 8. PMID: 31912754.

[45] Lan A, Lee A, Munroe K, McRae C, Kaleis L, Keshavjee K, Guergachi A. Review of cognitive behavioural therapy mobile apps using a reference architecture embedded in the patient-provider relationship. Biomed Eng Online. 2018 Dec 17;17(1):183. DOI:10.1186/s12938-018-0611-4. PMID: 30558610; PMCID: PMC6296144.

[46] Hannah Maria Jennings, Joanna Morrison, Kohenour Akter, Abdul Kuddus, Naveed Ahmed, Sanjit Kumer Shaha, Tasmin Nahar, Hassan Haghparast-Bidgoli, AK Azad Khan, Kishwar Azad & Edward Fottrell (2019) Developing a theory-driven contextually relevant mHealth intervention, Global Health Action, 12:1, DOI:10.1080/16549716.2018.1550736

[47] Schroé H, Van Dyck D, De Paepe A, Poppe L, Loh WW, Verloigne M, Loeys T, De Bourdeaudhuij I, Crombez G. Which behaviour change techniques are effective to promote physical activity and reduce sedentary behaviour in adults: A factorial randomized trial of an e-and m-health intervention. International Journal of Behavioral Nutrition and Physical Activity. 2020 Dec;17(1):1-6.

[48] Milne-Ives M, Lam C, De Cock C, Van Velthoven MH, Meinert E. Mobile Apps for Health Behavior Change in Physical Activity, Diet, Drug and Alcohol Use, and Mental Health: Systematic Review JMIR Mhealth Uhealth 2020;8(3):e17046 DOI:10.2196/17046

[49] Jiang L, Liu S, Li H, Xie L, Jiang Y. The role of health beliefs in affecting patients' chronic diabetic complication screening: A path analysis based on the health belief model. J Clin Nurs. 2021 May 5. DOI:10.1111/jocn.15802. Epub ahead of print. PMID: 33951248.

[50] Abuzinadah AR, Alanazy MH, Butt NS, Barohn RJ, Dimachkie MM. Exacerbation Rate in Generalized Myasthenia Gravis and Its Predictors. Eur Neurol. 2021;84(1):43-48. DOI:10.1159/000512077. Epub 2020 Dec 15. PMID: 33321491; PMCID: PMC7969373.

[51] Paglialonga A, Patel AA, Pinto E, Mugambi D, Keshavjee K. The healthcare system perspective in mHealth. In m_Health current and future applications 2019 (pp. 127-142). Springer, Cham. DOI:10.1007/978-3-030-02182-5_9

[52] Chib A, Lin SH. Theoretical advancements in mHealth: A systematic

review of mobile apps. Journal of health communication. 2018 Nov 2;23(10-11):909-955.

[53] J. Geuens, L. Geurts, K. Gerling, R. D. Croon and V. V. Abeele, "A Dyad of Lenses for the Motivational Design of mHealth: Bridging the Gap between Health Theory and App Design," 2019 IEEE International Conference on Healthcare Informatics (ICHI), 2019, pp. 1-12, DOI:10.1109/ICHI.2019. 8904839.

[54] https://www.lensesofmotivational design.com/ accessed May 11, 2021.

[55] Babich, N., 2021. A Comprehensive Guide To Mobile App Design [online] Smashing Magazine. Available at: <https://tinyurl.com/bc4xv4be> [Accessed 11 May 2021].

[56] Brommels M. Patient Segmentation: Adjust the Production Logic to the Medical Knowledge Applied and the Patient's Ability to Self-Manage-A Discussion Paper. Front Public Health. 2020 May 27;8:195. DOI:10.3389/ fpubh.2020.00195. PMID: 32537449; PMCID: PMC7267007.

[57] Read, L., & Korenda, L. (2019, October 29). How do consumers navigate the health care frontier? Deloitte Insights. Available at: https:// tinyurl.com/3bpcspfz [Accessed May 10, 2021].

[58] Riihimies R, Kosunen E, Koskela T. Web-Based Patient Segmentation in Finnish Primary Care: Protocol for Clinical Validation of the Navigator Service in Patients With Diabetes. JMIR Res Protoc. 2020 Nov 2;9(11):e20570. DOI:10.2196/20570. PMID: 33136062; PMCID: PMC7669435.

[59] Sandy R, Connor U. Variation in medication adherence across patient behavioral segments: a multi-country study in hypertension. Patient Prefer Adherence. 2015 Oct 29;9:1539-48. DOI:10.2147/PPA.S91284. PMID: 26604707; PMCID: PMC4631417.

[60] Masud, Mohammed T., et al. "Unobtrusive monitoring of behavior and movement patterns to detect clinical depression severity level via smartphone." Journal of biomedical informatics 103 (2020): 103371.

[61] Arora, Siddharth, et al. "Detecting and monitoring the symptoms of Parkinson's disease using smartphones: A pilot study." Parkinsonism & related disorders 21.6 (2015): 650-653.

[62] Rajalakshmi, Ramachandran, et al. "Automated diabetic retinopathy detection in smartphone-based fundus photography using artificial intelligence." Eye 32.6 (2018): 1138-1144.

[63] Taylor, James A., et al. "Use of a smartphone app to assess neonatal jaundice." Pediatrics 140.3 (2017).

[64] Cartledge S, Maddison R, Vogrin S, Falls R, Tumur O, Hopper I, Neil C. The utility of predicting hospitalizations among patients with heart failure using mHealth: Observational study. JMIR Mhealth Uhealth. 2020 Dec 22;8(12):e18496. DOI:10.2196/18496.

[65] Yim SJ, Lui LMW, Lee Y, Rosenblat JD, Ragguett RM, Park C, Subramaniapillai M, Cao B, Zhou A, Rong C, Lin K, Ho RC, Coles AS, Majeed A, Wong ER, Phan L, Nasri F, McIntyre RS. The utility of smartphone-based, ecological momentary assessment for depressive symptoms. J Affect Disord. 2020 Sep 1;274:602-609. DOI:10.1016/j.jad.2020.05.116. Epub 2020 May 25. PMID: 32663993.

[66] Shin KE, Newman MG, Jacobson NC. Emotion network density is a potential clinical marker for anxiety and depression: Comparison of ecological momentary assessment and

daily diary. Br J Clin Psychol. 2021 May 7. DOI:10.1111/bjc.12295. Epub ahead of print. PMID: 33963538.

[67] Radhakrishnan K, Kim MT, Burgermaster M, Brown RA, Xie B, Bray MS, Fournier CA. The potential of digital phenotyping to advance the contributions of mobile health to self-management science. Nurs Outlook. 2020 Sep-Oct;68(5):548-559. DOI:10.1016/j.outlook.2020.03.007. Epub 2020 May 8. PMID: 32402392.

[68] Gharani P, Karimi HA, Syzdykbayev M, Burke LE, Rathbun SL, Davis EM, Gary-Webb TL, Mendez DD. Geographically-explicit ecological momentary assessment (GEMA) architecture and components: Lessons learned from PMOMS. Inform Health Soc Care. 2021 Feb 20:1-20. DOI:10.1080/17538157.2021.1877140. Epub ahead of print. PMID: 33612061.

[69] Yang YS, Ryu GW, Choi M. Methodological Strategies for Ecological Momentary Assessment to Evaluate Mood and Stress in Adult Patients Using Mobile Phones: Systematic Review. JMIR Mhealth Uhealth. 2019 Apr 1;7(4):e11215. DOI:10.2196/11215. PMID: 30932866; PMCID: PMC6462888.

[70] Juengst SB, Terhorst L, Nabasny A, Wallace T, Weaver JA, Osborne CL, Burns SP, Wright B, Wen PS, Kew CN, Morris J. Use of mHealth Technology for Patient-Reported Outcomes in Community-Dwelling Adults with Acquired Brain Injuries: A Scoping Review. Int J Environ Res Public Health. 2021 Feb 23;18(4):2173. DOI:10.3390/ijerph18042173. PMID: 33672183; PMCID: PMC7926536.

[71] Gallacher KI, Quinn T, Kidd L, Eton D, Dillon M, Elliot J, Johnston N, Erwin PJ, Mair F. Systematic review of patient-reported measures of treatment burden in stroke. BMJ Open. 2019 Sep 18;9(9):e029258. DOI:10.1136/bmjopen-2019-029258. PMID: 31533946; PMCID: PMC6756342.

[72] Cerimele JM, Goldberg SB, Miller CJ, Gabrielson SW, Fortney JC. Systematic Review of Symptom Assessment Measures for Use in Measurement-Based Care of Bipolar Disorders. Psychiatr Serv. 2019 May 1;70(5):396-408. DOI:10.1176/appi.ps.201800383. Epub 2019 Feb 5. PMID: 30717645; PMCID: PMC6543835.

[73] Alappattu M, Harrington SE, Hill A, Roscow A, Jeffrey A. Oncology Section EDGE Task Force on Cancer: A systematic review of patient-reported measures for sexual dysfunction. Rehabil Oncol. 2017 Jul;35(3):137-143. PMID: 29082117; PMCID: PMC5656275.

[74] Stewart VM, Mendis MD, Low Choy N. A systematic review of patient-reported measures associated with vestibular dysfunction. Laryngoscope. 2018 Apr;128(4):971-981. DOI:10.1002/lary.26641. Epub 2017 May 23. PMID: 28543184.

[75] White DK, Master H. Patient-Reported Measures of Physical Function in Knee Osteoarthritis. Rheum Dis Clin North Am. 2016 May;42(2):239-52. DOI:10.1016/j.rdc.2016.01.005. Epub 2016 Mar 17. PMID: 27133487; PMCID: PMC4853650.

[76] Dias N, Boring E, Johnson LA, Grossoehme DH, Murphy S, Friebert S. Developing a theoretically grounded, digital, ecological momentary intervention for parental bereavement care using the ORBIT model-phase 1. Death Stud. 2021 Apr 29:1-10. DOI:10.1080/07481187.2021.1914239. Epub ahead of print. PMID: 33913789.

[77] Hawker CO, Merkouris SS, Youssef GJ, Dowling NA. A Smartphone-Delivered Ecological Momentary Intervention for Problem Gambling (GamblingLess: Curb Your Urge): Single-Arm Acceptability and

Feasibility Trial. J Med Internet Res. 2021 Mar 26;23(3):e25786. DOI:10.2196/25786. PMID: 33769294; PMCID: PMC8088874.

[78] Lucas-Thompson RG, Rayburn S, Seiter NS, Broderick PC, Smyth JM, Coatsworth JD, Henry KL. Learning to BREATHE "Plus": A Multi-Modal Adaptive Supplement to an Evidence-Based Mindfulness Intervention for Adolescents. Front Public Health. 2020 Nov 17;8:579556. DOI:10.3389/fpubh.2020.579556. PMID: 33282814; PMCID: PMC7705247.

[79] Carroll, L., 2021. Experimental phone app works with insulin pumps to control diabetes [online] Reuters. Available at: <https://tinyurl.com/9yk8bce8> [Accessed 11 May 2021].

[80] Hawker CO, Merkouris SS, Youssef GJ, Dowling NA. A Smartphone-Delivered Ecological Momentary Intervention for Problem Gambling (GamblingLess: Curb Your Urge): Single-Arm Acceptability and Feasibility Trial. J Med Internet Res. 2021 Mar 26;23(3):e25786. DOI:10.2196/25786. PMID: 33769294; PMCID: PMC8088874.

[81] Blevins CE, Marsh EL, Stein MD, Schatten HT, Abrantes AM. Project CHOICE: Choosing healthy options in coping with emotions, an EMA/EMI plus in-person intervention for alcohol use. Subst Abus. 2020 Sep 1:1-8. DOI:10.1080/08897077.2020.1806182. Epub ahead of print. PMID: 32870129.

[82] Nugent NR, Pendse SR, Schatten HT, Armey MF. Innovations in technology and mechanisms of change in Behavioral interventions. Behav Modif. 2019 Apr 29:145445519845603. DOI:10.1177/0145445519845603. Epub ahead of print. PMID: 31030527.

[83] Nice.org.uk. 2021. Overview | Evidence standards framework for digital health technologies | Guidance | NICE [online] Available at: <https://www.nice.org.uk/corporate/ecd7> [Accessed 11 May 2021].

[84] Ninds.nih.gov. 2021. Myasthenia Gravis Fact Sheet [online] Available at: <https://tinyurl.com/5ctyf2cc> [Accessed 11 May 2021].

[85] Goldenberg, W. and Sinert, R., 2021. Emergent Management of Myasthenia Gravis: Overview, patient history, physical examination [online] Emedicine.medscape.com. Available at: <https://tinyurl.com/5jzd7kfc> [Accessed 11 May 2021].

[86] Wolfe GI, Herbelin L, Nations SP, Foster B, Bryan WW, Barohn RJ. Myasthenia gravis activities of daily living profile. Neurology. 1999 Apr 22;52(7):1487-1489. DOI:10.1212/wnl.52.7.1487. PMID: 10227640.

[87] Lee I, Kaminski HJ, McPherson T, Feese M, Cutter G. Gender differences in prednisone adverse effects: Survey result from the MG registry. Neurology-Neuroimmunology Neuroinflammation. 2018 Nov 1;5(6).

[88] Keer-Keer T. The lived experience of adults with myasthenia gravis: A phenomenological study (Doctoral dissertation, University of Otago).

[89] McCarthy, J., 2019. One in five U.S. adults use health apps, wearable trackers [online] Gallup.com. Available at: <https://tinyurl.com/2spvu4we> [Accessed 11 May 2021].

[90] Ryan, Richard M.,Deci, Edward L. (2000). Self-determination theory and the facilitation of intrinsic motivation, social development, and well-being. American Psychologist, 55(1), 68-78

[91] Beshears J, Kosowsky H. Nudging: Progress to date and future directions. Organ Behav Hum Decis Process. 2020 Nov;161(Suppl):3-19. DOI:10.1016/j.obhdp.2020.09.001. Epub 2020 Dec 10. PMID: 33716395; PMCID: PMC7946162.

Section 2

A Discourse on Smart and Pervasive Health

Chapter 4

Emerging from Smoke and Mirrors

Lo Fu Tan

Abstract

Digital Health promises to transform healthcare in this decade. We have gone from "low tech" telephones, fax machines, dictation lines, desk-top electronic medical records, and data storage centers to video visits, texting, emails, smart phones and other mobile devices, and to higher forms including artificial intelligence, cloud data storage, and blockchain. However, letting go of legacy applications and then implementing the best available technology for clinical use has been challenging. This chapter will review the factors that contribute to the difficulty of moving from old to new tools. Specific examples will be video, electronic medical records and remote patient monitoring. The process of evaluating a new technological application will be described and a standardized framework proposed. We will finish with a discussion around local and scaled steps that can facilitate, support and sustain a patient-centered application of the best technology in healthcare. A call to action for the reader will be presented.

Keywords: digital tools, accessibility criteria, evaluation, implementation, strategic goals

1. Introduction

The experience of Healthcare is not pleasant. Accessing and navigating the system to receive timely care of high quality and affordable is not easy for patients. Cumbersome operational processes and inefficient legacy tools cause clinicians to waste time and promote burnout. Stakeholders- including payers and members, clinicians and their patients, industry, government agencies, and non-profit organizations- crave for a new paradigm that is smooth, seamless, and individualized. In 2020, technology was heralded as the means to make this happen by an end-to-end and fully integrated approach—all in a timely fashion under a viable business model that is cost-effective.

Despite the diversity of priorities amongst stakeholders, they can share a singular vision around technology. Digital Health, synonymous with Technology in Healthcare, is commonly defined as a convergence of digital technologies with Health, Healthcare, living, and society [1]. Furthermore, the author's vision of Digital Health- a patient-centered application of the best available technology to further the Quadruple Aim of better patient experience, clinician engagement, affordability, and quality [2]- can undoubtedly be adopted by all users of Healthcare. The technology we are talking about are just tools to make Healthcare easier for everyone but always starting and finishing with the patient.

What is facilitating this drive for the digitalization of Healthcare? As a practicing family physician for over 35 years, this author believes that the phenomenon is mostly due to our inability to meet demand requirements. The general practitioner had it right by providing in-person care in the office or emergency department or hospital or home, wherever the patient needed it. This clinician knew the patient well due to 1:1 clinical encounters and continuity through follow-up, so it was very personalized. Care was relatively affordable as testing and treatment, and referrals and appointments were decided based more on the clinical necessity and less on profit and liability. However, the shortage of primary care physicians, even with nurse practitioners and physician's assistants, has resulted in the erosion of this relationship and the gold standard of care. Virtual ways of communicating and "seeing" patients, although not ideal, are practical and can help.

Even with the coronavirus pandemic, the healthcare system has kept consumer engagement a top priority though some would argue for the wrong reasons such as sustaining and growing membership. Many capabilities have been strained and changed, but on a positive note, Digital Health has been pushed to the forefront with its promise of being able to have a positive impact on Healthcare, care delivery, and, ultimately, health. At the beginning of 2020, we were doing national presentations on audiovisual visits to promote the value of this type of care, especially for those with poor access. In 2019, only 11% of US consumers had used telehealth, but this has skyrocketed to 46% in 2020 [3]. We all experienced the rapid adoption and growth of telemedicine out of necessity due to ambulatory care and hospital facilities limiting access, and reduced utilization from fear of exposure while at brick and mortar settings. Those with an established video care component had modest increases from 2019 to 2020. In our urgent care telemedicine clinic, which has been in existence since 2013, volume tripled, or increased year to year by 200%. Nevertheless, clinical groups who had done limited video care pre-pandemic saw unprecedented exponential growth. In our multispecialty practice, both primary and specialty care divisions had nearly a 20,000% increase year to year.

An audiovisual connection was unquestionably the most prominent example of a Digital Health tool used during this crisis. There are many others. Texting applications, especially around symptom-checkers, were introduced. Some focused on mental health for those that could do self-care. Surgical centers found excellent use to reduce physical contact with patients during pre-operative management and post-operative follow-up. In direct response to the pandemic, Covid-19 symptom checkers were distributed by CDC, individual payers, and provider groups. Employers have also been using customized versions for employee wellness and surveillance.

These are some of the countless technological tools that the health care system is deploying to improve the patient experience end-to-end. This effort preceded the pandemic, but it has become even more critical as direct, in-person contact is of clinical concern. The historical exponential growth of Digital Heath in the technology industry accelerated in 2020 to unprecedented levels. It is much like the dot com era. Start-ups and established companies are professing to have the "solution" to a health care problem or case use through their software or "system" or "model." Worldwide in 2018, there were 318,000 mobile apps and 200 new ones per day [4]. These numbers have grown exponentially ever since.

A huge challenge for leaders in dealing with Digital Health is to figure out which technological tools to select. They have to decide if a device or application can perform as advertised. It is essential to determine if it will have an impact on the quality of care and outcomes. Affordability is always a concern too. Also, consideration must be given to legacy applications – are they worth keeping and integrating with the new? Or should they just be retired? While the first step is to find a reliable and reproducible way to identify Digital Health solutions of high quality and value, a framework for implementation is essential.

The myriad of stakeholders may share a high sense of urgency about Digital Health, but each has distinctive priorities that make all of this difficult to put into practice. We need to try to move Digital Health hopes systematically from "smoke and mirrors" to impactful reality if we are to create a truly better healthcare experience and system for all. In this chapter, let us look at the challenges of the initial selection of technological solutions. Then we will introduce a scorecard as a good starting point for evaluating the technology's quality. Next, a methodology is presented to measure outcomes. Finally, we will offer barriers to implementation, then some suggestions for a strategic framework.

2. The challenge

Dr. Eric Topol, who many consider being the father of modern Digital Health, presents Artificial Intelligence as a solution to make Healthcare human again. In his book Deep Medicine, he describes how technology can do this but warns that it will be a "marathon without a finish line." He points out that this is mostly due to inadequacies of AI technology, both functionally and from the lack of evidence-based clinical outcomes [5]. This scarcity of proof is the main reason why healthcare decision-makers are reluctant to invest in the resources to evaluate and use new Digital Health technologies. Lim and colleagues did a survey of CEOs from start-ups regarding slow healthcare adopters to digital technology. All agreed that this was due to the asymmetric impact of regulatory pressures; that is, even if a Digital Health product met regulatory requirements, healthcare providers were reluctant to accept risk as there was no evidence to support outcomes. Another reason was the need for multidisciplinary buy-in from other stakeholders [6].

Cost issues due to prior investment and ongoing maintenance of existing technological applications likely play a role. Most organizations have not done reliable cost analysis studies. When we have looked at this informally within our national organization, retiring legacy applications that were not needed or not useful lead to substantial overall one-time and annual cost savings even with the added expense of new solutions.

To illustrate the current "standard" evaluation process, we want to share three examples of technology used in our practice. These are not unique as there are many similar scenarios in other healthcare systems. Video for direct patient care is spotlighted since the pandemic has pushed it to the forefront. We have had urgent care video visits for years. Still, our established platform was not easy to apply in specific case uses- poor connectivity in hospital and home, difficulties for the patient to create an account, benefit confirmation, and navigating the application. The offshoot has been superficial and informal evaluation then rapid implementation of many other video platforms. Well-intentioned champions lead these on a case-by-case needs basis, and none were adequately studied. The result is a host of video applications, multiple contracts, patient and clinician confusion and frustration over many duplicate tools. The "back up" applications (which some intentionally use as their primary ones) are meant for social media and not safe medical use. We have quadrupled the number of video applications in our multispecialty group, and there does not appear to be an end in sight. The approach is straightforward: solve the problem in isolation, and no matter what device is needed, get it, and put it into production.

Another example centers on getting more value out of video visits. These typically do not include vital signs, exam modalities, and post-visit testing like a laboratory. We have an in-house kit that has been used for years to do remote patient monitoring on chronic patients like those with congestive heart failure. It contains blue-tooth enabled tools and a phone-linked tablet. The patient takes their blood pressure, weight, oxygen saturation, pulse, and temperature, with results automatically uploaded from the tablet to the company's web dashboard. We have modified it to meet our episodic need for vital signs before a scheduled video visit or to follow labile patients like those with uncontrolled hypertension over a few days. The patient can efficiently perform self-directed vital signs, uploaded to the provider's Medical Assistant, who then transcribes the data to the patient's EMR. A phone call then connects the patient at the pre-arranged time for the kit's video visit.

Concurrently, two other tablet devices are being tested by our national provider organization even though the first tablet with the Blue-tooth enabled vital signs tools appears much easier for the patient and physician to use. These other two do not have Bluetooth-enabled vital signs tools, so manual ones are delivered simultaneously as the tablet. We are currently comparing the three devices, but this is not being done in a formal, systematic way. An important point here is that the delivery means and organizational process, cleaning, and repacking are similar no matter the device used. The cost of the tool and how it performs are the main differentiators. Of course, politics too. One of our sister care delivery organizations has seen excellent results using one of these devices in engaging seniors at home and at the curbside, which has led to significant gap closure of population health measures. An outside vendor is offering this one. The other two belong to our company, which means a financial impetus to develop new case uses.

Another company's video option is the cheapest via a supplemental monthly physician subscription fee, easiest to scale, and already shown to work well. We have used their core function of texting between providers for years. They quickly developed secure, compliant, and high-quality connectivity to patients via texting and audiovisual, which allowed many case uses, including visits with patients in Skilled Nursing Facilities (SNIFs), home, and the curbside. It is as simple as texting the patient with an invitation to connect for an audiovisual visit on their smartphone or other connected devices. Naysayers question whether or not patients have access to their own devices capable of reliable audiovisual connectivity. Our surgical centers have been using this and have found that 75% of seniors have reliable personal mobile phones. We are still piloting three tablets, which are more expensive, not as easy to use, and possibly not scalable.

Our care delivery organization has had an Electronic Medical Record (EMR) program for nearly 20 years. With the overall goal of improving communication between patients and colleagues, we have contracted with the EMR vendor to add other components of a patient management solution- a patient portal, a program for scheduling, and video and texting applications. Another national vendor has the video platform that we have used for many years. It, too, is quickly adding other communication modes- texting and a stand-alone mobile video application. While both vendors appear to have solutions for comprehensive virtual care and communication, we have not been afforded the chance to test them. There also have been limited learnings from real clinical settings. Much of the vendors' offerings are still being developed. Even if a preliminary look is optimistic, we will have to spend time and money on further development and testing to end up with a final customized tool.

We recently started a pilot looking at a third option. A global tech company has a comprehensive communication tool that is easy to use, inexpensive, and customizable. We are looking to see if it can streamline connectivity between clinicians and staff, improve patients' experience doing video visits and scheduling, and allow easy connection to patients in the community. For example, hospitalized patients need a discharge "navigator" to coordinate care and follow-up and better medication adherence through real-time reconciliation to reduce Emergency Department visits and re-admissions. We are facing two stumbling blocks with testing- lack of access to the full functionality of the software and no workforce dedicated to conducting most pilot components.

What drives a tool's incorporation into a trial or pilot? It should always begin with a clinical or health care need or problem, or a case use that a technological tool or solution can help. Next, the device must meet all "Availability Criteria"- technologically sound- meaning that it works the way it professes to, is easy to use, is scalable, is customizable, and is affordable. Now it could move on to the pilot step for testing in a live environment. These examples of devices have not met the necessary criteria but are in pilots or have already been put into use.

Subjective business decisions made in isolation are often the culprit. The goal of getting to one EMR across many provider groups is appropriate. However, technology leadership is singularly focused on this directive and not properly vetting the vendor's ability to deliver and support the tool's capabilities, functionality, and need for development. Deadlines are missed, and costs are exceeded. Still, worst of all, the solution may never get to intended production.

We have many corporate leadership examples, seeing "the next best thing to come in Digital Health." A tool is quickly given capital support from the company or is acquired. Advocates demand quick implementation of the device. Often, it has no explicit end-user use, has not passed the five Availability Criteria, nor has it been shown to improve outcomes in formal pilots.

We see this coming from many other non-clinical divisions. The marketers who have historically been given Digital Health leadership roles love tools to enhance patient experience via the internet. The technology leaders find or create tools that they can solve problems with from their technological perspective. Neither group engages much with clinicians to determine their initiatives' implications on patients, providers, care, and outcomes.

So, we do not have an excellent way to evaluate the technology. Validation requires that we study the technology and potential outcomes. First, though, a problem is identified as the reason for trying out the technological solution.

Case uses can be about a specific problem or very broad. They can be for clinical or non-clinical. Short-term or long-term. Patient-specific or physician-specific. Provider System or Payer. It is easy to add in others. **Table 1** illustrates some examples. These case uses should be compatible with the vision and strategic goals of Digital Health and the overall organization.

Case Use	End User		
	Patient	Physician	Payer
Easy communication	X	X	X
Improved medication adherence		X	
Reduce ED utilization and readmission	X	X	
Front-end connection to system			X
Appropriate specialty referrals		X	X
Reduced EMR clicks		X	
Real-time data for CDS		X	
Shared data	X	X	X

Table 1.
Examples of end-use requirements or case uses.

3. Validation of digital health

Any method should take into consideration all five of the Availability Criteria of a technological tool. The Global Score of Mathews and his colleagues shows promise. The authors have completed a thorough review of the current state of validation of Digital Health. They feel that stakeholders have low confidence in Digital Health solutions due to a lack of an objective way to evaluate products. They propose an end-user requirements approach assessment across the four technological, clinical, usability, and cost domains. Their Digital Health Scorecard incorporates these four criteria, which they aggregate into a composite Global Score. We are presenting this as a means to determine the gross initial selection of Digital Health solutions. Individual scores can allow sufficient discrimination of particular products, identify where improvements are needed or gaps, and compare similar Digital Health solutions [7]. Focusing on a few is imperative as resources are usually scarce.

The Global Scorecard uses a multi-stakeholder approach that purportedly can objectively and rigorously evaluate solutions. It is comparable to methodologies used outside of Healthcare (such as Underwriter's Lab, which develops safety standards and uses pre-market testing, and Consumers' Reports, which relies on post-market evaluation). It appears flexible and dynamic enough to meet the demands of multiple stakeholders. For example, payers want more efficient use of resources, whereas providers want increased reimbursement. The current scorecard uses end-user requirements to determine the maximum impact on patients. This approach can be transparent, thorough, and standards-based [8]. It is currently being tested for validity in different studies.

4. Quadruple aim-based outcome measures

A formal pilot to assess technology is essential before a full launch. Measures of outcomes need to be created to determine how well the solution performed, especially regarding helping solve the problem for a specific case use. From the author's Digital Health vision to help achieve the Quadruple Aim, let us see how we might use this to formulate our outcome measures. Dr. Don Berwick and his colleagues introduced the Triple Aim to improve the patient's care experience and populations' health and reduce costs to improve the US Healthcare System [9]. This evolved into the Quadruple Aim as the importance of caring for the provider was acknowledged. Many health care organizations have adopted the four aims as their overarching goals. There has never been an impetus to rank them. However, without patients, the health care system would have no reason to exist. Even if quality and patient satisfaction are outstanding, cost-prohibitive care and a lack of clinicians or staff due to low engagement will lead to a model that could not be sustained. The prevailing priority is to improve the patient and clinician experience, hopefully leading to better clinical quality and cost control.

Concerning patient satisfaction, surveys are the means to collect data. Overall, questions are not specific enough, so we need more directed ones that tie back to case uses. Patients are now also customers and consumers. They want to interact with the health care system as they see fit, not just by the traditional telephone call and in-person visit, which involves a process that is not easy to use. They want to engage using virtual tools like audiovisual connections, texting, and e-mailing. They want to be able to self-schedule. They want to get referrals, tests, results, and prescriptions quickly. Price transparency is essential too. Finding tools that can achieve these wishes is our mandate.

Physician Engagement starts with ways to improve the EMR so that there are fewer clicks, less need for brain power and time, and better workflows. Frustration over the EMR has directly contributed to the burn out of providers and staff who are less caring and less careful, directly impacting the patient experience and clinical care quality. There is less attrition of patients, physicians, and staff when they are satisfied and engaged. Human capital groups agree that it costs nearly $1 M to replace a physician throughout the healthcare system. We do not know the effect of turnover on patient satisfaction and quality of care, but both are likely reduced.

Quality in Medicine has always been about clinical criteria- the quality of life, reduced morbidity, and reduced mortality. The Quadruple Aim's focus, however, is on the overall health of the population. Historically, this was under the purview of Public Health and Preventive Medicine but has morphed into its own Population Health discipline. Measures created by government agencies in collaboration with payers, provider groups, and academic institutions are geared towards payment and are only indirect measures of quality of life, morbidity, and mortality.

Cost considerations have evolved over the years, going from dollars adjusted for inflation to Cost-Effectiveness to Return on Investment to Medical Waste calculations. Value-based care, coupled with Evidence-Based Medicine as a core component of decision-making, has gained enormous popularity since it is a useful cost control model. The hope is that this approach will significantly impact the estimated 1/3 of all medical costs being spent unnecessarily in the USA.

For any of the four Quadruple Aim goals, investigators can create specific outcome measures for a pilot. Financial Analysts must choose newer and more innovative ways to factor in non-monetary benefits. For example, engagement leads to better care, less morbidity and mortality, less attrition of patients and providers and staff, more retained, and new patients. A surrogate measure might be non-productive patient time for travel, waiting, and going to the pharmacy. Alternatively, for a physician, measure time to chart in the EMR, lost productivity due to missed appointments from no-shows, and face-to-face time with a patient.

5. Letting go

Letting go of legacy applications or figuring out how to integrate them with new technology is a challenge. Our leadership contracted with the EMR vendor with minimal clinician input. Over the years, albeit not unlike most EMR applications, it has not come close to meeting our providers' and staff's expectations. It is not agile nor easily customizable. Only one user can get full functionality on a patient chart at any one time, although a workaround has allowed for limited simultaneous access. It takes multiple clicks to complete a repetitive task, like entering an electronic prescription. Most frustrating for all is that the responsiveness from the vendor to technological issues is insufficient. In part, our organization is responsible for this since we decided to have extensive home-grown IT and CAS groups to manage this EMR for customization and cost-saving. The result forces the clinician to work for the computer rather than the computer working for the clinician. Despite these concerns, it has become the go-to EMR in our region. This vendor has also entered into the patient management product lane by introducing its patient platform, a scheduling application, and patient communication solution, including video and texting. This process has been three years in the making, but out-of-the-box baseline functionality is low, and much of their solution requires ongoing development.

There are practical concerns about retiring this EMR. We have used it for nearly two decades, and moving to another may not make things better. The cost of starting over is a primary issue. Another important consideration is that the ends justify the means- going to a single or limited number of EMRs in a region makes sense from data access and sharing perspectives, and cost. Doing this without making sure that the product meets all five Availability Criteria- does the technology do what it professes? Is it easy to use? Customizable? Scalable? Cost reasonable?- makes no sense. An appropriate comparative analysis looking at other EMR products should be done. Considering novel approaches such as a front-end wrapper might be worthwhile. Foundational applications from companies with such expertise are more likely to be readily available and not require the cost and time of development we are experiencing.

Letting go also encompasses the siloed approach to Digital Health that has plagued organizations for years. Modern-day Digital Health began its foray into health care 20 years ago with marketing teams looking at the internet and consumers. These groups continue to champion customer experience and end-to-end service. They work diligently to use technology to connect with consumers and patients to receive an outstanding experience similar to other thriving service industries. While they do look at end-user requirements or case uses, these are typically non-clinical. Technology groups do the same from their narrow application perspective. Success for them is in the implementation of a solution and making it work based on technical specifications. Again, consideration of clinical end-user requirements is often an afterthought. Business and financial groups do similar isolated Digital Health work to get data for operational efficiency reasons. Both payers and providers have marketing, technology, business, and finance divisions doing comparable work in their parallel silos. Finally, the payers and the clinical groups look at Digital Health from their relatively narrow perspectives. If all of these groups could collaborate and communicate effectively, share tools and data and resources, and agree on end-user requirements or use cases, we would be much further ahead in achieving practical evaluation and implementation of Digital Health tools.

6. Implementation: towards a strategic plan

Mathews and his colleagues address organizational factors by suggesting that there is no single owner of a Digital Health solution requirement, making it challenging to come up with a scorecard that all would embrace. They state that there are no known optimal requirements due to so many new Digital Health applications. It is hard to determine which stakeholder should take ownership of driving the requirements. We propose that the lead be a blended payer-provider one. This dyad could fulfill the role of the primary owner. Cogan et al. suggest that a collaborative effort between a payer and provider for health IT can be successful by sharing tools and tactics leading to technological systems' interoperability, agreeing on clinical goals and quality measures of outcomes, and sharing data from standard quality measurement tools [10].

A dyad ought to follow these recommendations.

Operationally, Mathews and colleagues feel that it is not practical to vigorously evaluate more than a few Digital Health solutions at a time, which makes a scorecard more justifiable for high-cost conditions or those in peer-reviewed studies for validation purposes. They wonder if the industry should not self-evaluate. How likely will they take this on as it would be both expensive and time-consuming? Do any of the other stakeholders want this coming from the industry instead of a more objective source?

Mathews et al. correctly propose that what is essential for the future are resources, collaboration, and time to validate the Digital Health Scorecard and needing input from all stakeholders to align financial incentives to outcomes appropriately. They propose that governmental regulatory bodies and provider health systems lead this. However, they point out that nontraditional players may do better, e.g., CVS and Aetna, Amazon-JP Morgan Chase-Berkshire Hathaway. Even so, these entities are missing knowledge and experience from a critical group, the clinicians.

Stotz et al. interviewed a group of "Next-Generation Payer and Providers (NGPPs)" who have payers and clinicians collaborating effectively: Alignment Healthcare, Clover Health, CareMore Health, Iora Health, and Oscar Health. These payers have new payment models that redefine how patients interact with their health plans. Providers or clinicians are on value-based payment models, engaged in upstream clinical monitoring, focused on primary care, and committed to population health. These NGPPs consider technology to be the key enabler of their innovative approaches, including predictive analytics, price and outcome transparency, on-demand care via telemedicine, and AI for care decisions. Key learnings from these NGPPs: use technology to enable more person-to-person interaction, either co-develop or buy from the technology company but not both, use real-time data to support decision making, consider Remote Patient Monitoring for home-based care but know that the technology is not currently easy to use and validation is lacking, and give consideration to creating beta-testing clinic sites for pilots [11].

Any implementation framework should include the concurrent evaluation of existing and new technological applications for specific case uses. An end-user requirements approach and a combined Global Score, followed by a Quadruple Aim-based outcome analysis, is ideal. The result would be a set of data-driven recommendations for review.

The final decision regarding tool selection should be made easier by the process I have described. Who will make this determination? As we are using these technological tools to solve problems that span Health and Healthcare, the input from multiple stakeholders would be invaluable- Digital Health, Technology, Marketing, Finance, Medical Management, Population Health, Legal, Human Resources, Patient Experience, Providers and Payers. All parties should have been involved from the beginning and through to the end of this collaborative effort. A consensus supported recommendation would go to an "executive board" made up of the Digital Health business and clinical leaders, CMIO, CMO, and CEO for final ratification. Evidence-Based Medicine (EBM) is an excellent model to follow, in which the best available research evidence forms the core of medical-decision making. However, EBM is not perfect since we lack good research evidence for the testing and treatment standards of many of the medical problems we face. In part, this is why we have a pyramid from a base of little evidence that uses expert opinion in the form of guidelines up to the peak with meta-analyses.

So, where does this leave us? Recall that Evidence-Based Medicine is not just about the best available research findings. David Sackett reminds us that it must include the addition of clinician experience and the patient's input [12]. This is consistent with Medicine being an art. That collaboration between patient and physician is a crucial component. The process of technological tool evaluation is similar. It is also an art that uses facts based on Digital Health Scorecard results, Quadruple Aim-based measures to assess pilots' outcomes, and the best available experience, then getting input from all stakeholders for the best decision.

Evaluation of the technology is about the standards to follow for the innovation and change that will come as part of an overall Digital Health strategy. Other strategic goals directly impact standards and need to encompass organizational and operational leadership and governance, investments, and workforce. There should be a means to approve and conduct pilots across different ecosystems while providing advisory and consultation support. Digital Health leadership would have much input into the sustainability, spread, and scaling of successful innovations.

Selecting a method for evaluating Availability Criteria, then the value of a tool through Quadruple Aim-based outcome measures is a vital strategy responsibility. Collaboration with clinical partners in the organization to get buy-in to positively affect workflows, time, expenses, and integration, while dealing with unintended consequences, e.g., expectations regarding higher standard of experience with virtual communication. Leadership would have input into payment model design for new care models to improve the patient experience while meeting both payer and provider financial expectations. A key role would be to formulate a plan to place technological applications into the community for population health interventions. The strategy should look at the social determinants of health to use technology to alleviate those detrimental factors to access and clinical outcomes.

There are no excellent established value and impact-based business models for Digital Health. Next-Generation Payers and Providers (NGPP) may be a good starting point since a provider stakeholder is directly involved. These companies were created to deliver a re-imagined service to patients, prioritizing health, and outcomes over utilization. The onus is not placed on the consumer or patient. The payer and the provider have direct risks and ultimately share responsibility for the customer and patient's health and care and Healthcare.

As a starting point, any Digital Health's strategy should consider short-term goals for both the consumer and the stakeholders. We all want our members and patients to have convenient, safe, effective virtual care. Both payers and providers see the value in doing a better job at managing chronic conditions, improving medication adherence, and reducing unnecessary emergency department visits and hospital admissions. Focusing on the elderly and the poor and the disadvantaged racial groups and those social determinants negatively impacting health is vital. Directing patients toward timely and appropriate care at the right location can begin today. Finally, we can use Digital Health tools to facilitate looking after the whole person's overall health [13].

Drury et al.'s working paper on investing in Digital Health provides a guide on how to think about the process. It can help put together the data needed to allow for a well-informed investment decision through the Digital Health Impact Framework (DHIF Appendix 2 pp. 56–59). The DHIF includes a list of crucial questions for each stakeholder to consider:

1. What is the social and political context? Is there the will and finance to pursue a good case through to implementation?

2. What are the options, including possible public-private partnerships?

3. Do the options fit with health, health care, and Digital Health strategies?

4. What are the intended and probable results, and how long will it take to realize them?

5. What are the priority investments planned, their cost, and how do they help achieve the intended and probable results? This stage can make use of modeling tools for assessing cost and benefits over time and should address: (i) How and when will benefits be realized; (ii) Required results of the preferred option that has the highest priority to be achieved; (iii) Estimated costs and benefits for each stakeholder type; (iv) Estimated monetary values of the benefits; (v) Socio-economic returns for each option and their adjustments for sensitivity, optimism bias, and risk exposure; (vi) How risks will be mitigated; (vii) How and where services will be delivered; (viii) Focus of services; and (ix) Life cycles, affordability of options.

6. What are the priority actions within the resources available?

7. How will the results be monitored and evaluated?

In building the investment case, it will be important to show that:

i. The proposed initiative is needed and fits well with other relevant strategies.

ii. It represents value for money.

iii. It is commercially viable.

iv. The main investors, who may not be the direct beneficiaries, can afford it.

v. It is achievable.

A means to measure, monitor, and improve performance is mandatory. The Digital Health Impact Framework's (DHIF) consistent methodology provides an appraisal of estimated costs, benefits, net benefits, the socio-economic returns, and financial affordability over time of individual digital health projects. It enables bespoke appraisals that can be aggregated to help leaders and planners to:

(i) Understand and develop the socio-economic and financial aspects of their digital health strategies, modify them as needed, and (ii) Make informed investment decisions for sustainable digital health programs and projects.

DHIF is a proven methodology used in over 60 evaluations. It starts by setting a timeline that broadly matches an investment's life cycle. Then, researchers can prepare assumptions and estimates of types of users and stakeholders for each year. DHIF should include estimated changes from Digital Health projects, such as healthier citizens and communities, and more appropriate health care utilization. These arise from Digital Health's impact on patients, care providers and citizens, health workers, and health care organizations.

Drury et al. also propose that for any implementation to be successful, while leadership is the key, investment is necessary. This investment must come with clear justification by understanding the context and process for such investment decisions. Success also depends on better data management, including integrating and sharing data, agreement on policies and standards, good security, and all stakeholders getting needed resources. They felt that most digital health investment decisions would do well financially concerning affordability and return on investment and support the workforce population's overall productivity in general.

Here are the important components for strategy from Drury et al. [14] (Author comments have been added):

Leadership and governance- (to identify the preferred leadership and governance model), the collaboration between clinical and business sectors is vital. We favor a dyad that would direct strategic planning and implementation. Each partner comes with unique training, experience, knowledge, and skills to positively impact the Digital Health program. However, governance must include other stakeholders: payer, clinicians, patients, technology, marketing, finance, and patient experience. Success depends on full collaboration and cooperation, which must be a high priority and responsibility of these two leaders who have authority at an executive and enterprise-wide level.

Strategy and investment- (to produce a description of the Digital Health strategy and investment components required to support the development and operation of the program) Drury et al. have four key focus areas which we believe should guide all strategic and investment goals:

1. Foundations- Digital Health components that will allow the sharing of information/data.

2. Solutions- Digital Health components that access and interact with, and use foundations to access and share information.

3. Change and Adoption- motivate and support the health system, establish incentives, and identify changes needed in work practices.

4. Governance- coordination, visibility, structures, and mechanisms for accountability and effective leadership.

5. The strategy includes developing a business plan to justify and follow progress that is built-in. It needs to include a framework for where to start, what technology to evaluate, and how to do this, an implementation plan, resource and workforce needs, and associated costs. Sustainability must be considered- what is needed to maintain and upgrade, re-evaluate, conduct ongoing pilots, adjust to innovation, and change strategy. Ongoing evaluation is required, which demands executive authorization of resources for all stakeholder groups.

6. Services and application- (to produce a description of Digital Health service and application components required to deliver outcomes described by the initial vision) Need to decide who should maintain the technology and who should deliver and support the clinical service. Delivery of the clinical service needs to be addressed.

7. Infrastructure- (to produce a description of Digital Health infrastructure components required to support Digital Health services and application components). You need to select a connectivity platform from an established technology company with resources and know-how.

8. Standards and Interoperability- (to support Digital Health service and application, infrastructure, and health information flows). The current chapter's focus.

9. Legislation, Policy, and Compliance- (to produce a description of Digital Health legislation, policy, and compliance components required to develop and operate the Digital Health program) Cyber-security is vital.

10. Workforce- (to produce a description of the Digital Health workforce required to develop, operate, and support the Digital Health program) skilled and matrix management ready.

7. Conclusion

"Smoke and Mirrors" aptly describes the current state of Digital Health. To make it smart and pervasive, we need a way to validate Digital Health tools. Start with a particular case use or problem needing a technological solution. Next, using a Global Scorecard, determine if Availability Criteria are met. See if it genuinely helps the case use or end-user requirement by conducting a pilot to report outcome measures from the Quadruple Aim. Using an implementation framework within the context of an overall Digital Health strategy led by a payer-physician dyad, a formal set of findings and recommendations can be presented to executive leadership. All are charged with supporting the final decision as a Digital Health program's success depends ultimately on taking timely and appropriate action.

Acknowledgements

To Sharon Manarin and Matthew Tan for their support of this project.

Conflict of interest

None.

Author details

Lo Fu Tan
Southwest Medical Associates, Nevada, United States of America

*Address all correspondence to: lo-fu.tan@optum.com

References

[1] Digital Health Solutions Bringing a 'Health Experience .... https://consultqd.clevelandclinic.org/digital-health-solutions-bringing-a-health-experience-revolution/

[2] Bodenheimer T, Sinsky C. From triple to quadruple aim: care of the patient requires care of the provider. Ann Fam Med. 2014 Nov;12(6):573-576.

[3] Bestsennyy O, Gilbert G, Harris A, Rost J. Telehealth: a quarter-trillion-dollar post-COVID-19 reality? McKinsey and Company, Healthcare Systems, and Services. May 29, 2020.

[4] Liquid State. The Rise of mHealth Apps: a market snapshot. https://liquid-state.com/mhealth-apps-market-snapshots/ (2018).

[5] Topol E. Deep Medicine. How Artificial Intelligence Can Make Healthcare Human Again. Basic Books, Hachette Book Group. New York. 2019.

[6] Lim SY, Anderson EG ICCSS'16: Proceedings of the 2016 49th Hawaii International Conference on System Science (HICSS) January 2016 Pages 3328-3337.

[7] Mathews SC, McShea MJ, Hanley CL, Ravitz A, Labrique AB, Cohen AB. Digital Health: a path to validation. NPJ Digit Med. 2019 May 13;2:38. DOI: 10.1038/s41746-019-0111-3. eCollection 2019.

[8] Mathews SC, McShea MJ, Hanley CL, Ravitz A, Labrique AB, Cohen AB. Reply: Some considerations on digital health validation. NPJ Digit Med. 2019 Oct 17;2:103. DOI: 10.1038/s41746-019-0176-z. eCollection 2019.

[9] Berwick DM, Nolan TW, Whittington J. The triple aim: care, health, and cost. Health Affairs 27, no.3(2008):759-769.

[10] Cogan S. How payers and providers can align and collaborate, with and without vertical integration. Health IT Answers, Oct 29, 2020.

[11] Stotz c, Zweig M. Next-generation payers and providers: setting a strategy for tech-enabled innovation. The Rock Weekly Rock Health 2020.

[12] Sackett DL, Rosenberg WMC, Muir Gray JA, et al. Evidence-based Medicine: what it is and what it isn't. BMJ 1996;312:71.

[13] Four Ways that Payers and Providers Can Collaborate on .... https://ramaonhealthcare.com/four-ways-that-payers-and-providers-can-collaborate-on-virtual-health/

[14] Drury P, Roth S, Jones T, et al. Guidance for investing in digital health. ADB Sustainable Development Working Paper Series. Asian Development Bank. No. 52 May 2018.

Section 3

Digital Platforms and Learning

Chapter 5

xCARE: A Development Platform for Supporting Smart and Pervasive Healthcare

Eloisa Vargiu, Meritxell Gómez-Martínez, Silvia Orte, Laura Ros-Freixedes, Kian Seif, David Marí and Felip Miralles

Abstract

We are assisting to an important change in the healthcare domain where healthy citizens and patients are more and more in the center and become active partners in the entire process. In this scenario, smart and pervasive solutions assume a relevant role for remotely assisting citizens and patients together with their carers and supporting the overall team of professionals. From a software-engineering perspective, to follow and/or anticipate changes in requirements, modular solutions must be investigated and developed. Moreover, issues like personalization, adaptation, and scalability must be considered from the very beginning. In this chapter, we present xCARE, a microservices-based platform explicitly implemented to support the development of smart and pervasive healthcare systems. To show the potentiality and adaptability of xCARE, three relevant applications are presented: (i) a self-management system to support chronic complex patients; (ii) a patient management system that allows the team of professionals to assist patients before a major surgery together with a self-management system for the patients themselves; and (iii) an automatic self-management system for healthy citizens that want to follow healthier habits and that supports behavioral change.

Keywords: development platform, microservices, software architecture, self-management system, complex chronic patients, health pillars, nutrition, sleeping, physical activity

1. Introduction

In the near future, healthcare has to rapidly move from a professional-centric system to distributed networked healthcare systems in which citizens become active partners in the entire healthcare process [1]. According to [2], there is the need to move from managing illness to managing wellness. In this new scenario, smart and pervasive healthcare plays an important role [3, 4].

Smart and pervasive healthcare refers to several different application fields: self-management of patients, health-status monitoring and follow-up, communication between patients and healthcare professionals, daily-life activities monitoring of citizens, as well as support for behavioral change for citizens of any age. The common perspective is assisting citizens remotely by relying on a set of sensors and/or devices (e.g., wearable and medical) suitably integrated together. In doing so,

IntechOpen

healthy people may adopt good habits and improve their overall wellness, whereas patients can be remotely assisted and improve their quality of life.

From a software-engineering perspective, developing smart and pervasive solutions for healthcare must take into account key issues such as personalization, adaptation, and scalability. In fact, developing robust monolith systems reached its limitations. Changes in requirements and implementation may imply that the systems evolve too slowly and inefficiently. Thus, a complex problem might be decomposed in easier sub-problems according to a divide-et-impera approach. In this direction, microservice architectures emerged and quickly became a widely used solution [5]. These architectures are especially appropriate for distributed environments in which several functionalities have to be provided separately or different sensors have to work together, as in the case of Internet of Things (IoT) solutions [6]. In this chapter, we propose a development platform, namely xCARE, suitably defined and implemented to give support in developing smart and pervasive healthcare systems. xCARE has been conceived in a very generic way in order to be adapted to any kind of scenarios. It has been built by relying on the concept of microservices. That approach has been adopted since microservices enable software to be divided into modules, making it easier to change and adapt it. In fact, microservices can be considered as modern agents that could improve systems in distributed environments [7].

The platform has been defined and developed as part of the CONNECARE H2020 project[1]. Thanks to its generic nature, it is also the baseline of the system currently under development in the PAPRIKA project[2], aimed at improving the quality of life and healthcare results of patients undergoing major surgery. Moreover, the IoT-based self-management system of the CarpeDiem project[3] has been built upon xCARE. Finally, xCARE is currently under adaptation for the eVisió project to give support to patients after an ophthalmic surgery[4].

After describing the overall platform and its main components, this chapter presents how xCARE has been used for: (i) providing self-management to complex chronic patients in the CONNECARE project, (ii) empowering and managing patients at home before a major surgery in the PAPRIKA project, and (iii) supporting behavioral change through a recommender system in the CarpeDiem project.

The remaining of the chapter is organized as follow. We present the xCARE platform in Section 2 and its adaptation for the CONNECARE, PAPRIKA, and CarpeDiem projects in Section 3. Section 4 sums up the main novelty of the approach comparing xCARE with other smart and pervasive platforms for healthcare. Finally, in Section 5, we end the chapter with some conclusions and lessons learnt.

2. A development platform for supporting smart and pervasive healthcare

xCARE is a platform that has been defined and implemented for supporting the development of smart and pervasive healthcare systems. It has been conceived in a very generic way in order to be adapted to any kind of scenarios. In fact, the "x" in its name means that it can be adopted and adapted for any application in the

[1] https: //www.connecare.eu/

[2] https://eithealth.eu/project/paprika/

[3] Funded by ACCIÓ Pla de Recerca i Innovació 2019/2020

[4] Compra Pública Innovadora or Pre-Commercial Procurement, co-financed by Fundació Salut Empordà and the Catalan Department of Health

healthcare field. xCARE can be easily customized and adapted to develop system for: patients' self-management; health-status monitoring and follow-up; allowing communication between patients and healthcare professionals; monitoring daily-life activities; integrating wearable- and medical-devices and gathering data from them; as well as giving recommendations and nudges to patients, citizens, and healthcare professionals to support behavioral change.

The microservice approach has been adopted since microservices enable software to be divided into modules, making it easier to change and to adapt it. **Figure 1** sketches the overall platform. It is composed of a set of microservices each of them in charge of performing a simple task. Complex tasks are achieved by the collaboration, interaction, and coordination of one or more simple microservice. In the Figure, connections between microservices are shown to point out those that cooperate together to reach complex goals. When changes are needed in a microservice, they do not affect the rest of the system. Moreover, when a new functionality is required, a new microservice (or a set of them) is defined and simply added to the system. In doing so, the proposed solution is robust to changes and improvements.

Each microservice is completely independent of the actual system that will use it. In this way, a set of microservices has been implemented and it is already available (e.g., for monitoring physical activities, for taking measurements from medical devices, for following up drug prescriptions). If the actual system needs one or more of the already-implemented microservices, it/they will be used "as is" as bricks to build the system. On the contrary, if the actual system needs to rely on a new functionality for which there is not a corresponding microservice, the new microservice will be defined from scratch in a very generic way to be used in the system and to leave it available in the generic xCARE platform for the development of further systems.

In order to locate the microservices, *Netflix-Eureka* service discovery is adopted [5]. Eureka is a REST based microservice for locating microservices with the purpose of load balancing and failover of middle-tier servers (the Eureka Server). Eureka also comes with a client component (the Eureka Client), which makes interactions with the microservice much easier. The client also has a built-in load balancer that does basic round-robin load balancing.

As a front door for all requests from the front-end and the microservices, we rely on *Netflix Zuul*[6]. Zuul is the front door for all requests from devices and websites to the backend of the Netflix streaming application. It is built to enable dynamic routing, monitoring, resiliency and security. It uses a range of different types of filters that enables to quickly and nimbly apply functionality to the edge microservice. These filters help performing the following functions: authentication and security, identifying authentication requirements for each resource and rejecting requests that do not satisfy them; insights and monitoring, tracking meaningful data and statistics at the edge in order to give an accurate view of production; dynamic routing, dynamically routing requests to different backend clusters as needed; stress testing, gradually increasing the traffic to a cluster in order to gauge performance; load shedding, allocating capacity for each type of request and dropping requests that go over the limit; and static response handling, building some responses directly at the edge instead of forwarding them to an internal cluster.

Management of roles, rights, authentication control, and login is implemented by relying on Spring Cloud Security[7]. It offers a set of primitives for building secure applications and services with minimum fuss; as well as a declarative model

[5] https://github.com/Netflix/eureka
[6] https://github.com/Ne5tflix/zuul/wiki
[7] https://cloud.spring.io/spring-cloud-security/

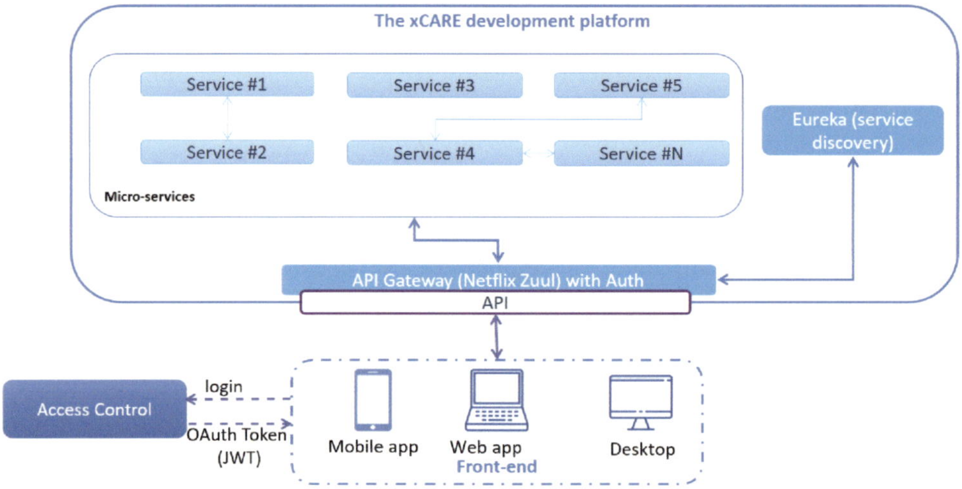

Figure 1.
The xCARE development platform at a glance.

which can be heavily configured externally (or centrally) and lend itself to the implementation of large systems of co-operating, remote components, usually with a central identity management service.

The front-end fully depends on the actual final system and the corresponding user-requirements and application. Different kinds of front-end can be developed: mobile apps, especially for patients, carers, or citizens who want to self-manage their status or activities; web apps, mostly for professionals that need to follow-up patients during an intervention; or desktop solutions to closed-system that need to directly interact to other systems, as for instance hospital information systems.

3. xCARE in action

Among the different implementations we have implemented and we are currently implementing by using xCARE as baseline, in the following, we present how xCARE has been used for providing self-management to complex chronic patients in the CONNECARE project and for supporting behavioral change through a recommender system in the CarpeDiem project.

3.1 Self-management of complex chronic patients

The project CONNECARE (Personalized Connected Care for Complex Chronic Patients) is a H2020 Research and Innovation Project, started on April 2016 and finished on December 2019. CONNECARE is a technologically-oriented initiative aiming at exploring digital tools to support two key requirements of integrated-care services for chronic patients, namely: (i) Smart adaptive case management of patients with multimorbid conditions; and, (ii) Collaborative work among the various stakeholders, including patients and their families across health and social care tiers, involved in the services. The CONNECARE approach uses an observational study design, focused on implementing the CONNECARE organizational model and technology in a real life clinical setting, with an intervention group and matched control group and four implementation sites: Barcelona and Lleida in Spain, Ashdod in Israel, and Groningen in The Netherlands.

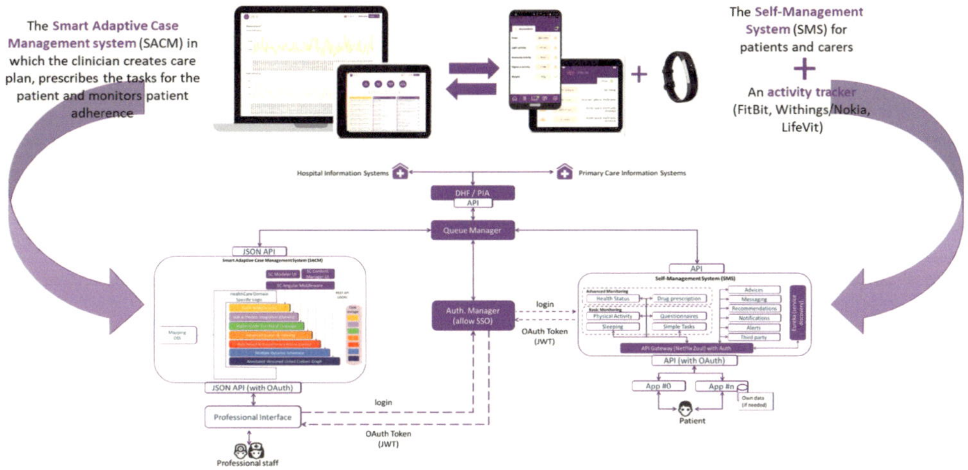

Figure 2.
The CONNNECARE overall system.

The CONNECARE system has been deployed in two situations: 1) Community-based prevention of unplanned hospital-related events in chronic complex patients with high risk for hospitalization; and 2) Preventive patient-centered intervention in complex chronic patients undergoing elective major surgical procedures. While the objectives and desired outcomes are the same in all sites, the organizational model for integrated-care and the supporting digital tools have been adapted to the specific needs of each site.

The CONNECARE system, depicted in **Figure 2**, is composed of a Self-Management System (SMS), installed on patients' smartphones (or tablets), and the Smart Adaptive Case Management system (SACM), accessible via Web. The SMS allows monitoring patients and providing engagement, rewards, and warnings [8]. The SACM has extended functionalities for case management to define a case according to an organizational model based on a 5-dimension score strategy: Case Identification, Case Evaluation, Workplan definition, Workplan execution, and Discharge [9]. Additionally, the SACM includes an advanced Clinical Decision Support System focused on helping clinicians in risk assessment and stratification and a visual support tool for locating the patients and organizing their visits [10]. The SMS and SACM interact each other through the CONNECARE Enterprise Service Bus which connects both subsystems and orchestrates their communication. All professionals, including health professionals from both primary care and hospitals and social workers, interact with each other using a direct communication tool to coordinate the patient's care plan and its execution, assuring continuity of care between hospital, primary-, and social-care. Patients continuously check their status and execute their assigned tasks through the SMS. Hospital staff, primary care professionals, and social workers may also help and accompany the patients using the messaging. CONNECARE provides also an integration framework to link its services to specific Electronic Health Records and regional Personal Health Folders.

The CONNECARE SMS has been built upon the xCARE platform. **Figure 3** sketches the adaption that has been done. In total, 12 microservices have been defined and developed, 7 of them specifically to perform patient's monitoring (5 for basic- and 2 for advanced-monitoring) and 5 are for giving support and providing further functionalities:

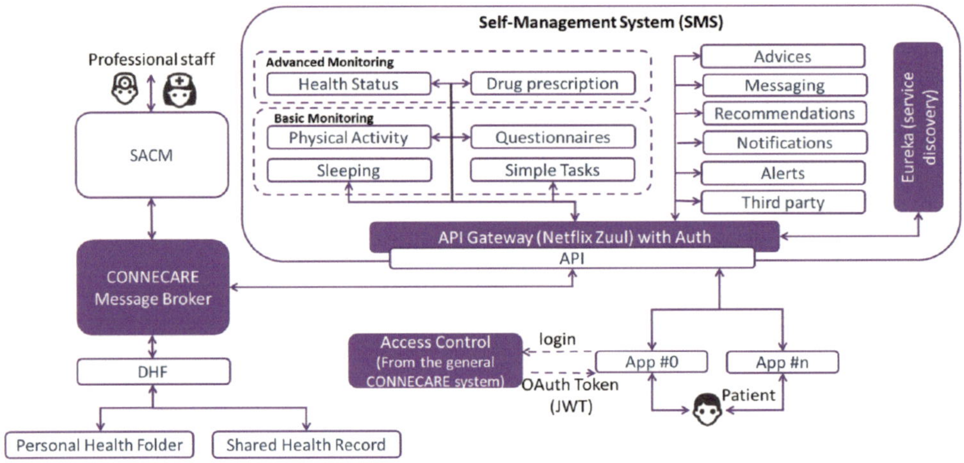

Figure 3.
xCARE adapted to CONNECARE.

- Basic Monitoring

    - Physical activity, to monitor the number of steps performed every day and the minutes of activity (low, medium, high, and sedentary). Wristbands from Withings[8] and Fitbit[9] have been integrated through the interaction with the corresponding APIs. Moreover, wristbands from LifeVit[10] have been directly integrated by relying to the Bluetooth connection.

    - Sleeping, to monitor sleeping data (sleep time per night, minutes that the user has been awake during the night sleep, and sleep time during the day) through the wristbands used for monitoring the physical activity.

    - Questionnaires, to assign one or more questionnaires to a patient; setting-up of the questionnaire(s) to be answered, together with the frequency that questionnaires will be requested to the patient's under the medical surveillance provisions; sending back questionnaire answers to the clinician; and checking the list of prescribed questionnaires and their answers.

    - Simple tasks, to monitor the performance of specific tasks during the day (e.g., dancing, cooking, reading). Moreover, depending on the disease and the kind of patient (e.g., in case of elderly people) the professional may ask to perform healthy activities such as drinking or eating a fruit. Through the self-management system, the patient can accept or reject the request and check when the activity has been performed.

- Advanced Monitoring

    - Health status, to monitor the health status of patients through the integration of suitable medical devices (e.g., blood-pressure monitor, thermometer, and pulse-oximeter). Devices from Withings have been selected because of the availability of the API and the possibility to ingrate

[8] https://www.withings.com/es/en/

[9] https://www.fitbit.com/

[10] http://lifevit.es/

them via Bluetooth or WI-FI. In case of traditional medical devices were preferred, also the manual input from the patients was allowed.

- Drug prescription, to remind to take a medication and to monitor the intake. Professionals prescribe all the drugs to be taken and the patient will receive a reminder any time s/he has to take one. In case of low adherence, a message is sent to both the patient and the professional.

- System

    - Advice, to allow professionals to select pieces of advice and training material in the form of text, images, or videos that patient is asked to see. The patient may create her/his own list of bookmarks to have a direct access to relevant information any time is needed. Four categories of advice have been defined: automatic advice (generated by the system according to the collected data), personalized advice (written by the professional for a specific patient), educational material (specific of a given case study in a specific site and common to all the patients of the corresponding case and site), and health educational videos (specific for a given site and common to all the patients to that site).

    - Messaging, to offer a bidirectional communication that allows patients to interact with members of the medical staff in charge of the case, a given clinician, or even with other patients or communities of patients. Similarly to the well-known Whatsapp app, patients may send/receive text, images, videos, links, and documents.

    - Recommendations, to send recommendations on physical activity [11].

    - Notifications, it receives the notifications generated by any of the other microservices whose recipient is the patient (e.g., a new prescription has been generated). Complex notifications coming from interaction with the patient's monitoring microservices may also be sent.

    - Alerts, as soon as a patient's monitoring microservice finds an anomaly, it interacts with this microservice and a suitable alert message is sent to both the patient (to be aware of the issue) and the clinical staff (to be informed and act accordingly). Anomalies are triggered any time the data gathered from the patient (e.g., through the medical devices or a questionnaire) exceeds a given threshold defined at prescription time (e.g., a critical heart rate value).

    - Third party, to integrate third party elements, such as wearable and medical devices. This microservice has two main functionalities: managing the connections to external providers and standardizing the data model.

A total of 301 patients have been involved. Satisfaction of patients and carers with the SMS has been evaluated by relying on the Likert Scales/Net-Promoter-Score [12] and the System-Usability-Scale[11]. Overall, the satisfaction was high, despite a significant number of challenges encountered along the way. Satisfaction was clearly linked to the perception that the SMS was part of an overall integrated-care process and the relationship between professionals and patients. Finally, the User eXperience analysis performed in Lleida (Spain) shows that, in order to

[11] https://www.usability.gov/how-to-and-tools/methods/system-usability-scale.html

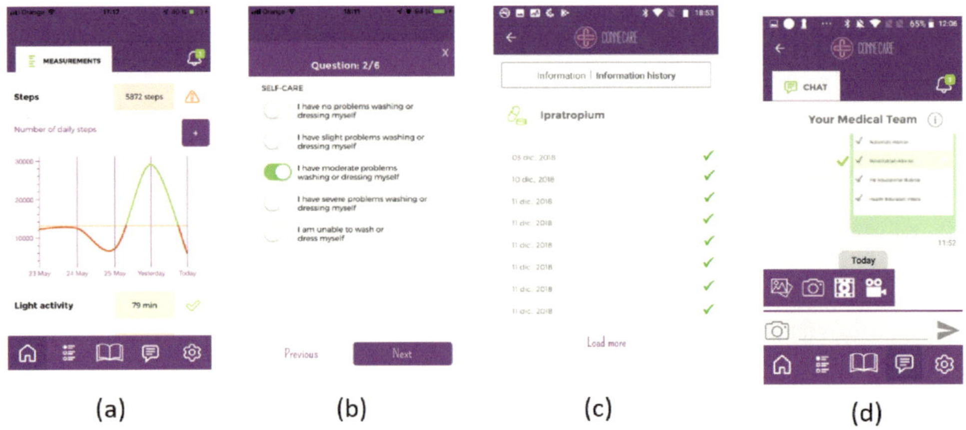

Figure 4.
Sample screenshots of the CONNECARE app showing: (a) the feedback on physical activity, (b) the administration of a questionnaire, (c) the follow-up of a drug prescription, and (d) the communications with the team of professionals.

improve satisfaction and engagement, patients need to perceive the app as relevant and that it gives them a clear and simple added value [13].

The CONNECARE SMS is an app available in both Apple App Store and Google Play markets[12]. **Figure 4** shows some screenshots of the CONNECARE SMS: (a) the feedback on physical activity in terms of number of steps, (b) the administration of the EQ-5D-5 L questionnaire, (c) the follow-up of the drug prescription of Ipratropium, and (d) the communications with the team of professionals showing the list of actions the patient may do.

3.2 Patient empowerment for major surgery preparation at home

The project PAPRIKA (patient empowerment for major surgery preparation at home) is an EIT Health Innovation Project, started in January 2019 and that will finish on January 2022. PAPRIKA establishes a technologically enabled and personalized program to prepare patients for elective surgery and to provide follow-up, as a way to improve the outcomes of the operation. The program develops close collaboration with the medical environment that empowers patients to co-create their own care. PAPRIKA will roll out its services fully in Spain, Germany, France, and Poland.

The project integrates short-term preoperative interventions, averaging about four weeks and including endurance training, promotion of physical activity and nutritional and psychological support. Interventions are planned both in the community and at the hospital, reducing unnecessary interactions between patients and tertiary care. The project incorporates two digital solutions (see **Figure 5**): a case management system for professionals, integrated with the electronic health record (EHR); and a self-management system for patients, integrated with the regional health folder. Both digital solutions have been built upon xCARE. **Figure 6** shows how xCARE has been adapted for the PAPRIKA aims. The following functionalities, powered by the xCARE microservice architecture, are currently available:

- Prescription, to allow professionals to prescribe any kind of tasks to the patients: physical activity, medical check-up, mindfulness and nutrition tasks, drug intake, and questionnaire filling.

[12] Apple store: https://apps.apple.com/es/app/connecare-h2020/id1364574255?l=en and Google Play: https://play.google.com/store/apps/details?id=connecare.mobile&hl=en

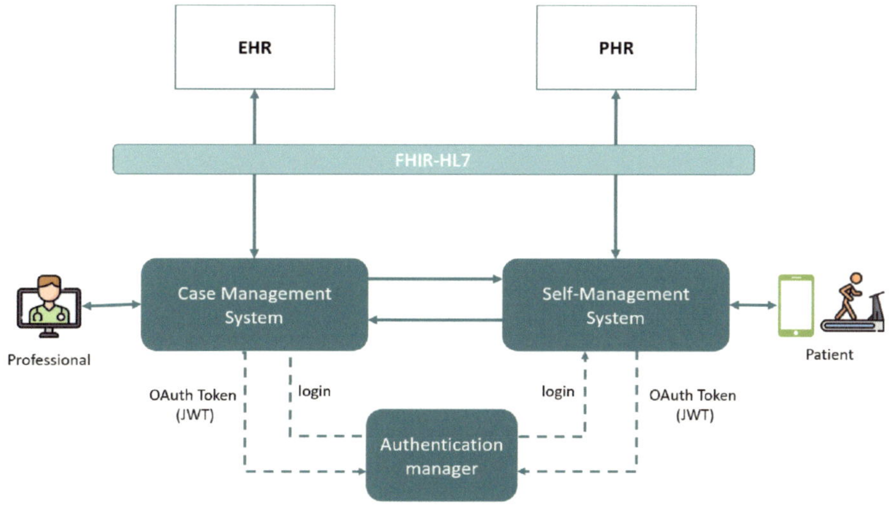

Figure 5.
A sketch of the PAPRIKA overall system.

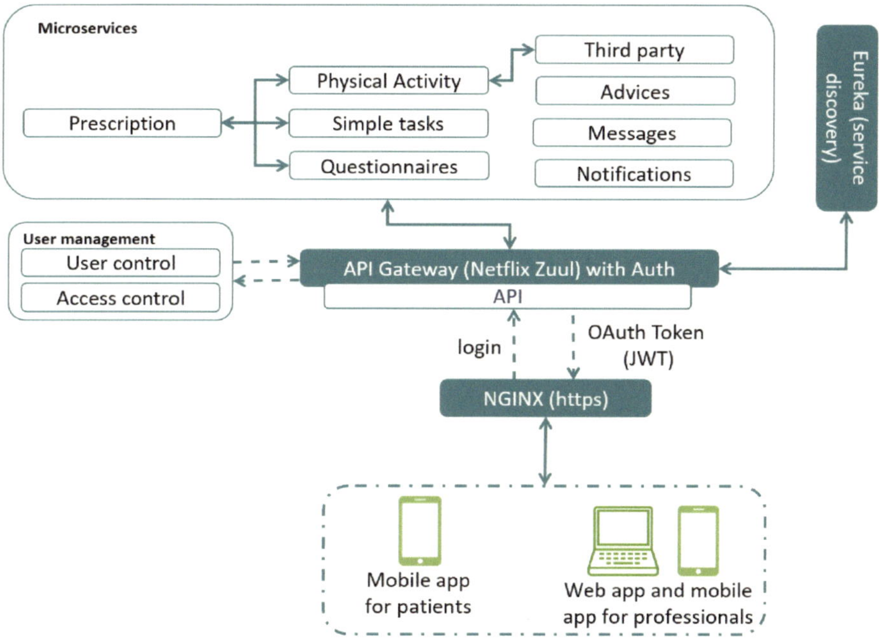

Figure 6.
xCARE adapted to PAPRIKA.

- Physical activities, to monitor the activities performed every day in terms of number of steps. Wristbands from Garmin[13] and LifeVit[14] have been directly integrated by relying to the Bluetooth connection.

- Simple tasks, to monitor the performance of specific tasks during the day related to nutrition habits (e.g., eat a fruit) or mindfulness activities (e.g., watch a given video).

---

[13] https://www.garmin.com/en-US/

[14] http://lifevit.es/

- Questionnaires, to assign one or more questionnaires to a patient, as for instance "how do you feel today?". The microservice then sends back the answers to the clinician.
- Third party, same behavior of CONNECARE.
- Advice, to send text, images, or videos containing suggestions or educational material to the patients. The pieces of advice are set-up an priori by the professionals and the patient may access them any time s/he needs.
- Messages, to offer a bidirectional communication that allows patients to interact with members of the medical staff in charge of the case, a given clinician, or even with other patients or communities of patients. Videocalls are also supported by this microservice.
- Notifications, to notify patients and professionals in case a microservice generates a notification or an alert (e.g., a prescription has been done, a new measurement has been taken, a questionnaire has been answered).

The pilot of PAPRIKA is currently running in the 4 sites (Spain, Germany, France, and Poland). The case management system for professionals is available in each hospital thanks to its integration with the EHRs, while the self-management system is an app available in both Apple App Store and Google Play markets[15]. **Figure 7** shows some screenshots of the case management system for the professionals: (a) the list of prescriptions of a patient; and of the self-management system for the patients (b) the main screen with the list of tasks to be performed, (c) the performed physical activity, and (d) the communications with the team of professionals in charge.

3.3 Collaborative and adaptive recommendations for personalized diet management

The project CarpeDiem (Collaborative and Adaptive Recommender for PErsonalized DIEt Management) is aimed at providing intelligent and automatic support to people who want to follow a diet to stay fit, lose or gain weight. The concept of "diet" in CarpeDiem is considered in an integral way, taking into account nutrition, physical- and sleeping-activity. CarpeDiem users are elderly people who need to follow a strict diet, athletes who want to control their weight and stay healthy or simply, people who want to follow a healthy diet.

CarpeDiem is an IoT-based intelligent self-management system aimed at monitoring physical- and sleeping-activity, nutrition, as well as environmental data and lifestyle habits, with the final goal of providing personalized recommendations and nudges to foster behavior change towards healthier behaviors [14]. The self-management system is bulit upon xCARE where intelligent techniques have been implemented for personalization and automatic monitoring, and a front-end is given in the form of an app to be installed in the citizen's smartphone.

As depicted in **Figure 8**, the IoT-based self-management system works with a set of data coming from different sources. CarpeDiem users wear an off-the-shelf activity tracker 24/7 to monitor physical- and sleep-activity as well as the energy expenditure in terms of calories. CarpeDiem users are also asked to monitor their weight once a week in order to take under control the Body Mass Index (BMI) and

[15] Apple store: https://apps.apple.com/us/app/prehab/id1466618747 and Google Play: https://play.google.com/store/apps/details?id=org.eurecat.prehab hl = es*MX*

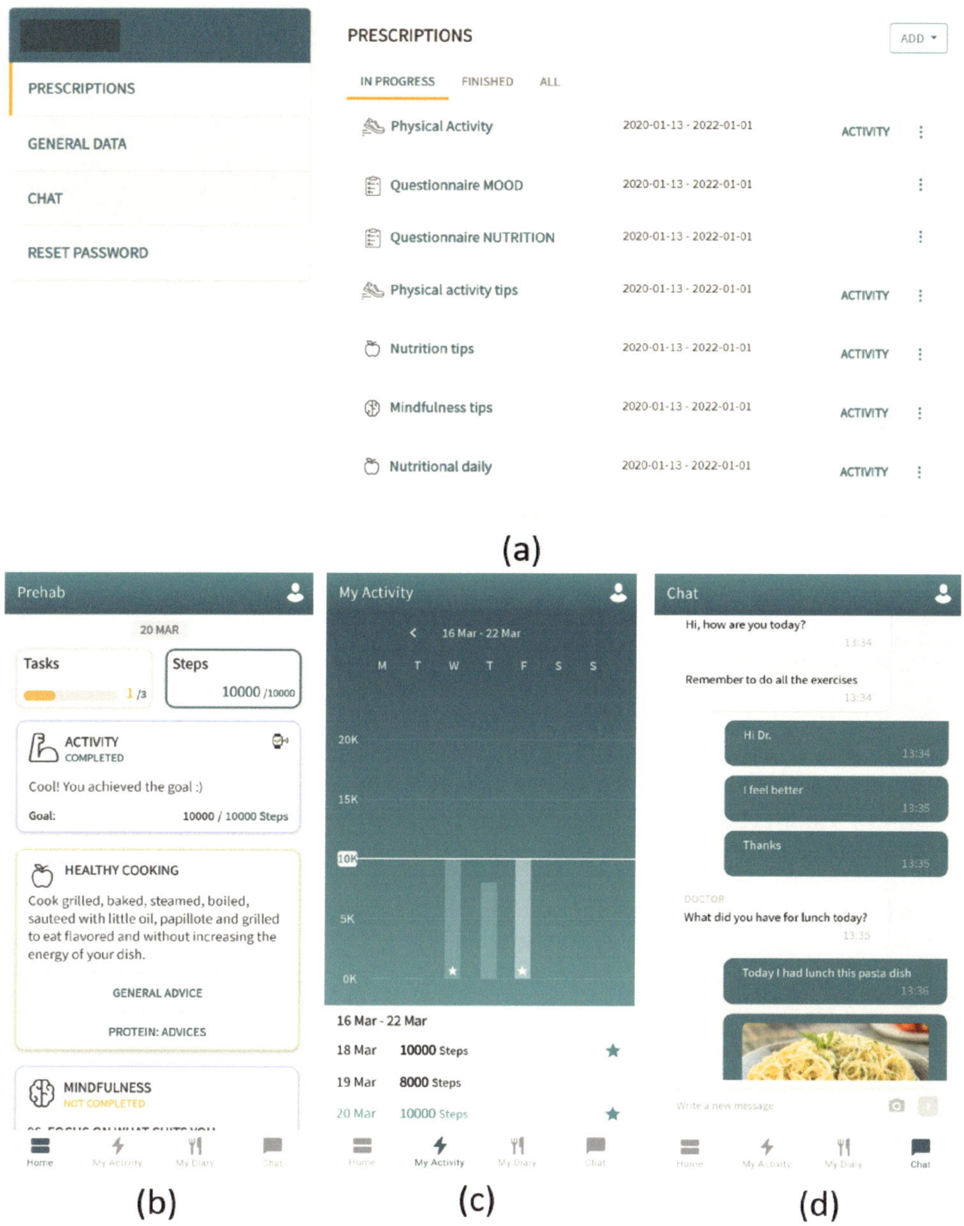

Figure 7.
Sample screenshots of the PAPRIKA digital tools showing: (a) the list of prescriptions assigned to a patient, from the case management system, and (b) the home screen with the list of activities to be performed today, (c) the performed physical activity, and (d) the communications with the team of professionals, from the self-management system.

to avoid reaching overweight and, thus, obesity. The CarpeDiem system integrates the LogMeal API [15], capable of recognizing meals through pictures taken from the smartphone camera. The pictures taken by using the CarpeDiem system are automatically sent to LogMeal that analyzes them and gives as output a list of meals. The citizen selects the right one and CarpeDiem automatically indicates the corresponding food group and calculates the number of calories and key nutrients of a dish portion, basing such calculation on the recipes also available through LogMeal. Moreover, questionnaires are used to directly ask the users regarding some lifestyle

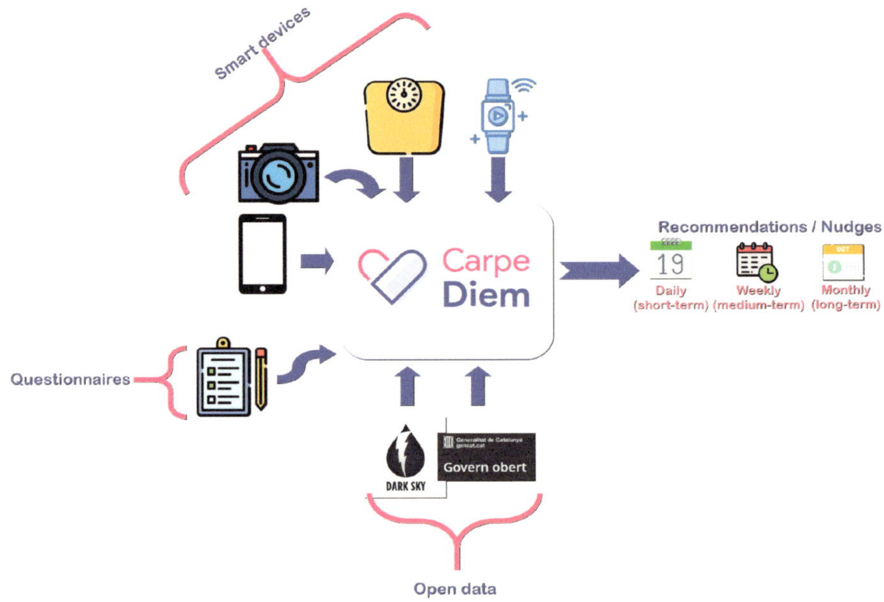

Figure 8.
The CarpeDiem IoT system at a glance.

habits. Finally, to be aware of the seasonality, the daylight hours, and further environmental data, we rely to the Dark Sky API[16], whereas to monitor the air quality (currently, only in Catalonia) Dades Obertes by Generalitat de Catalunya is used[17].

Figure 9 shows how xCARE has been adapted to implement the CarpeDiem IoT-based self-management system; 10 microservices have been implemented:

- Monitoring
    - Physical Activity, to monitor the walking activity by relying on an activity tracker.
    - Sleeping, through the activity tracker it automatically recognizes when the patient is sleeping or awake.
    - Nutrition, to monitor food intake by relying on the LogMeal app.
    - Weight, to monitor the increase/decrease of the weight by relying on a smart scale that automatically sends the data.
    - Questionnaires, to collect answers from the selected questionnaires: SATED [16], about the satisfaction of the citizen regarding her/his sleep; Smoke, on the number of cigarettes smoked on average during the week; Use of light-emitting screens, concerning the number of minutes spent on average using the smartphone or a tablet just before going to sleep; and Caffeine, to check the number of coffees, teas, and energy drinks the user drunk during the 7 hours before going to sleep, the day before.

[16] https://darksky.net/dev

[17] http://governobert.gencat.cat/en/dades_obertes/

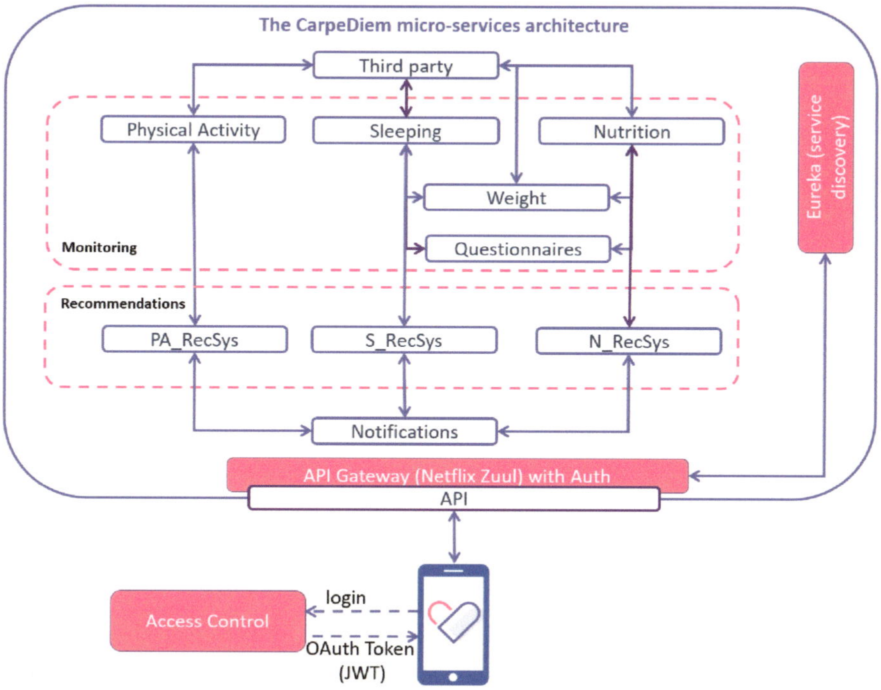

Figure 9.
xCARE adapted to CarpeDiem.

- Recommendations
    - PA_RecSys, according to the goal in terms of number of steps, it calculates the adherence day by day considering also the day of the week and the weather.
    - S_RecSys, analyzing the sleep habits gathering the information from the *Sleeping*, *Questionnaires*, and *Weight* microservices, it sends nudges and recommendations to follow better habits.
    - N_RecSys, generating the profile of the user, this service sends suggestions to change habits, as well as general recommendations on healthy foods.
- System
    - Third party, it implements the connections and calls the selected external APIs (i.e., activity trackers[18], smart scales[19], LogMeal, and open-data sources). This microservice works as an abstraction level. It only has to ask the third party connector for the information and wait for the data without worrying about the communication process and the different data model used.
    - Notifications, it sends to the front-end the notifications generated by any of the microservices.

[18] In the current version, we use activity trackers from Fitbit (https://www.fitbit.com/) and Withings(https://www.withings.com/) for monitoring steps, sleeping habits, and energy expenditure;
[19] In the current version, we use smart scales from Withings, for monitoring the weight and the BMI

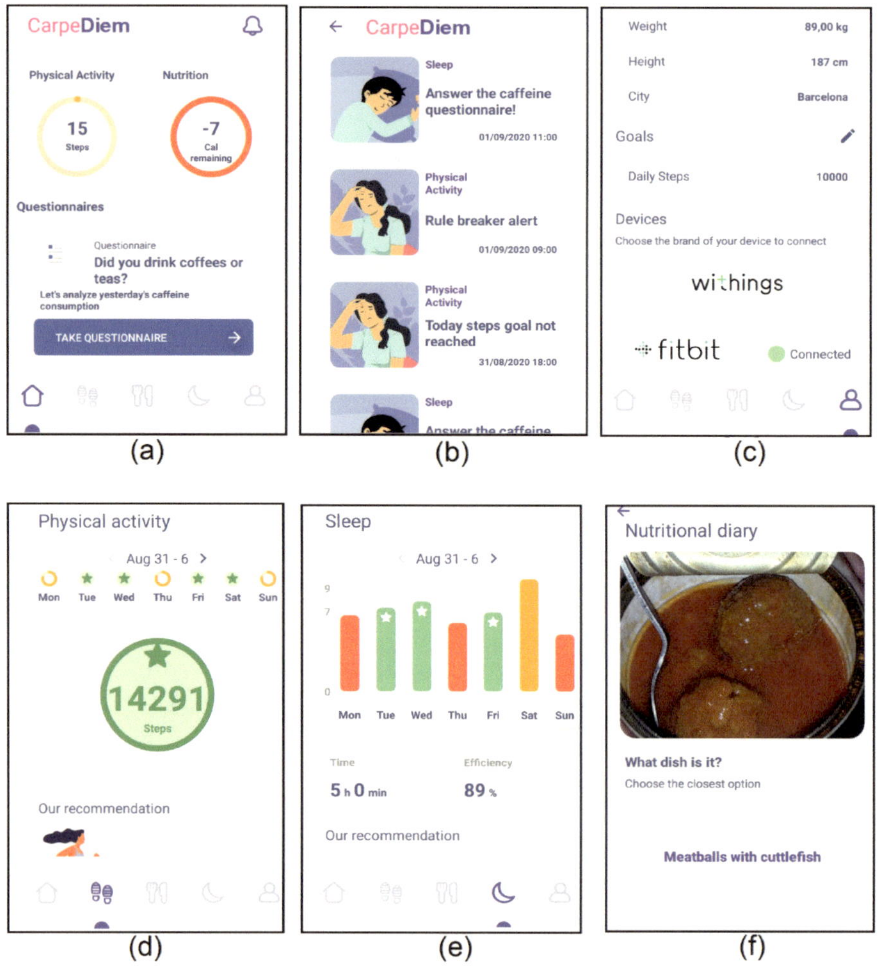

Figure 10.
The CarpeDiem app: (a) the main page with an overview of the activities; (b) a list of received notifications; (c) the setting page; (d) the physical activity details; (e) the sleeping activity details; (f) an example of food recognized from its picture.

The CarpeDiem IoT-based self-management system is an app available in the Google Play (early access) for Android smartphones[20]. On July 2020, a pilot started with 14 healthy volunteers recruited in Eurecat (35.64 ± 8.58 years old; 5 females; and 22.96 ± 2.67 BMI). The pilot, which will end at the end of the year, has a threefold objective: (1) collecting feedback to improve the app and/or correct bugs; (2) testing the usability and evaluating the user experience; and (3) gathering new data to improve the 3 recommender systems and start implementing the holistic one. Results of the pilot will be calculated in terms of usability once the pilot ends.

Figure 10 shows some screenshots of the Carpe Diem system: (a) the home page where the user has an overview of her/his status and may answer to the questionnaires; (b) a list of received notifications, each pillar represented by a different icon; (c) the setting page that shows, besides other information, that the app is linked to Fitbit; (d) the physical activity page with the summary of the steps per day and a green star indicating when the goal was achieved; (e) the sleeping page

[20] https://play.google.com/store/apps/details?id=com.eurecat.carpediem

with the summary of the current week showing the sleeping hours and the efficiency as calculated by Fitbit; and (f) an example of recognized food (meatballs).

4. Discussion

As described in Section 2 and then pointed out by presenting three relevant adaptations of xCARE in Section 3, the proposed platform can be easily customized and adapted to develop smart and pervasive healthcare systems. Our lessons learnt coming from the development and adoption of this generic architecture is that from a software engineering perspective the tasks to be done to develop a healthcare system are almost always the same as the functionalities to be provided. On the contrary, what changes from an application to another is related to personalization, usability, and intelligent support. This conclusion clearly supports the definition of a generic development platform, such as xCARE.

Thinking on the xCARE microservices as LEGO pieces, any new application can be built by composing them according to the requirements. Continuing with such metaphor, what differentiate each application is which pieces are used, how they are combined, their color, and the final aspect as a whole. Accordingly, first, a co-design approach should be performed involving the final users (at any level), domain experts (i.e., healthcare professionals), technicians, and user experience experts. In doing so, the specific front-end for that application will be designed and the usability issues will be taken into account at the very beginning. Once all the needs have been collected, the xCARE software engineer gathers the requirements, selects the microservices already available, defines those that are not, and designs the overall architecture. In parallel, the IoT programmers develop the interface for the connection with the required devices (if not already available) and the artificial-intelligent team defines the models for providing personalized and intelligent support to the final users.

It is worth noting that the adoption of this kind of solution is very effective for rapid prototyping, because the final users can have a first version available in very few time. Thanks to its modularity, the corresponding application is robust to changes in requirements, thus supporting application development in which different actors are involved. Finally, it can be scaled-up easily by simply adding new microservices/functionalities or by delegating tasks and functions to additional microservices.

5. Conclusions

This chapter presented the xCARE development platform suitably defined for smart and pervasive healthcare systems. The platform is currently adopted in several solutions adopted at the European level. To give a view of the potentiality of xCARE, three relevant projects in which the platform has been used have been presented.

As for the future work, we plan to improve the platform with more microservices, to enhance the intelligent support with further models based on artificial intelligence and to apply xCARE approach and technology to further healthcare domains and use cases.

Acknowledgements

CONNECARE (Personalized Connected Care for Complex Chronic Patients) was funded by the European Union's Horizon 2020 Research and Innovation Programme (under grant agreements nÂ° GA-689802).

CarpeDiem (Collaborative and Adaptive Recommender for PErsonalized DIEt Management) has been funded by ACCIÓ Pla de Recerca i Innovació 2019/2020.

PAPRIKA (Patient empowerment for major surgery preparation at home) has been funded by EIT Health Innovation BP2017.

Conflict of interest

The authors declare no conflict of interest.

Notes/thanks/other declarations

The authors would like to express their sincerest gratitude to all the patients that participated in the implementation studies of CONNECARE and all the volunteers currently testing the CarpeDiem system. We also want to thank all the developers of the system and in particular, Juan Manuel Fernández and Mauricio Gonzales-Gonzales for CONNECARE and Juan Ruiz Zaldivar for CarpeDiem and PAPRIKA. A great thanks also to all the CONNECARE and PAPRIKA consortia as well as the domain experts involved in CarpeDiem.

Abbreviations

BMI	Body mass index
CarpeDiem	Collaborative and Adaptive Recommender for PErsonalized DIEt Management
CONNECARE	Personalized Connected Care for Complex Chronic Patients
IoT	Internet of things
REST	Representational state transfer
SACM	Smart adaptive case management
SMS	Self-management system

Author details

Eloisa Vargiu*, Meritxell Gómez-Martínez†, Silvia Orte†, Laura Ros-Freixedes†, Kian Seif†, David Marí and Felip Miralles
Eurecat, Centre Tecnòlogic de Catalunya, eHealth Unit, Barcelona, Spain

*Address all correspondence to: eloisa.vargiu@eurecat.org

† These authors contributed equally.

References

[1] Korhonen, I., Parkka, J., Van Gils, M.: Health monitoring in the home of the future. IEEE Engineering in medicine and biology magazine **22**(3), 66-73 (2003)

[2] Dishman, E.: Inventing wellness systems for aging in place. Computer **37**(5), 34-41 (2004)

[3] Arnrich, B., Mayora, O., Bardram, J., Tröster, G.: Pervasive healthcare. Methods of information in medicine **49**(01), 67-73 (2010)

[4] Ng, J.K.Y., et al.: Ubiquitous healthcare: healthcare systems and applications enabled by mobile and wireless technologies. JoC **3**(2), 31-36 (2012)

[5] Namiot, D., Sneps-Sneppe, M.: On micro-services architecture. International Journal of Open Information Technologies **2**(9), 24-27 (2014)

[6] Vargiu, E., Zambonelli, F.: Agent abstractions for engineering iot systems: A case study in smart healthcare. In: Networking, Sensing and Control (ICNSC), 2017 IEEE 14th International Conference on. pp. 667-672. IEEE (2017)

[7] Krivic, P., Skocir, P., Kusek, M., Jezic, G.: Microservices as agents in iot systems. In: KES International Symposium on Agent and Multi-Agent Systems: Technologies and Applications. pp. 22-31. Springer (2017)

[8] Vargiu, E., Fernández, J.M., Gonzales-Gonzales, M., Morales-Garzón, J.M., Prunera-Moreda, K., Miralles, F.: A self-management system for complex chronic patients. International Journal of Integrated Care (IJIC) **19** (2019)

[9] Michel, F.: A Collaborative Purely Meta-Model-Based Adaptive Case Management Approach for Integrated Care. Ph.D. thesis, Technische Universität München (2020)

[10] Mariani, S., Vargiu, E., Mamei, M., Zambonelli, F., Miralles, F.: Deliver intelligence to integrate care: the connecare way. International Journal of Integrated Care (IJIC) **19** (2019)

[11] Fernández, J.M., Mamei, M., Mariani, S., Miralles, F., Steblin, A., Vargiu, E., Zambonelli, F.: Towards argumentation-based recommendations for personalised patient empowerment. In: International Workshop on Health Recommender Systems, co-located with ACM RecSys 2017 (2017)

[12] Reichheld, F.F.: The one number you need to grow. Harvard business review **81**(12), 46-55 (2003)

[13] Vargiu, E., Dorado, A., Massip, M., Gómez-Martnez, M., Torres, G., de Batlle, J., Miralles, F.: User experience in connecare: Results and lessons learnt in lleida. XPA & Health Communication (2) (2019)

[14] Góomez-Martínez, M., Orte, S., Ros-Freixedes, Laura, a.S.K., Vargiu, E.: Empowering the citizen in the main pillars of health by using iot. In: EAI HealthWear 2020. p. to appear (2020)

[15] Bolaños, M., Valdivia, M., Radeva, P.: Where and what am i eating? image-based food menu recognition. In: European Conference on Computer Vision. pp. 590-605. Springer (2018)

[16] Bentez, I., Roure, N., Pinilla, L., Sapiña-Beltran, E., Buysse, D.J., Barbé, F., de Batlle, J.: Validation of the satisfaction, alertness, timing, efficiency and duration (sated) questionnaire for sleep health measurement. Annals of the American Thoracic Society **17**(3), 338-343 (2020)

Chapter 6

VIGOR: A Versatile, Individualized and Generative ORchestrator to Motivate the Movement of the People with Limited Mobility

Yu Liang, Dalei Wu, Dakila Ledesma, Zibin Guo, Erkan Kaplanoglu and Anthony Skjellum

Abstract

Physical inactivity is a major national concern, particularly among individuals with chronic conditions and/or disabilities. There is an urgent need to devise practical and innovative fitness methods, designed and grounded in physical, psychological and social considerations that will effectively promote physical fitness participation among individuals of all age groups with chronic health condition(s) and/or disabilities. This research is dedicated to achieving **V**ersatile, **I**ndividualized, and **G**enerative **OR**chestrator (**VIGOR**) to motivate the movement of the people with limited mobility. Tai-Chi is a traditional mind–body wellness and healing art, and its clinical benefits have been well documented. This work presents a Tai-Chi based VIGOR under development. Through the use of *Helping*, *Pushing* and *Coaching* (HPC) functions by following Tai-Chi kinematics, the VIGOR system is designed to make engagement in physical activity an affordable, individually engaging, and enjoyable experience for individuals who live with mobility due to disease or injury. VIGOR consists of the following major modules: (1) seamless human-machine interaction based on the acquisition, transmission, and reconstruction of 4D data (XYZ plus somatosensory) using affordable I/O instruments such as Kinect, Sensor and Tactile actuator, and active-orthosis/exoskeleton; (2) processing and normalization of kinetic data; (3) Identification and grading of kinetics in real time; (4) adaptive virtual limb generation and its reconstruction on virtual reality (VR) or active-orthosis/exoskeleton; and (5) individualized physical activity choreography (i.e., creative movement design). Aiming at developing a deep-learning-enabled rehab and fitness modality through infusing the domain knowledge (physical therapy, medical anthropology, psychology, electrical engineering, biomechanics, and athletic aesthetics) into deep neural network, this work is transformative in that the technology can be applied to the broad research areas of intelligent systems, human-computer interaction, and cyber-physical human systems. The resulting VIGOR has significant potentials as both rehabilitative and fitness modalities and can be adapted to other movement modalities and chronic medical conditions (e.g., yoga and balance exercise; fibromyalgia, multiple sclerosis, Parkinson disease).

Keywords: deep learning, 4D experience, virtual reality, kinetics, active orthosis, physical inactivity

 IntechOpen

1. Introduction

1.1 Motivation

Physical inactivity, particularly among aging adults and home-bound individuals with chronic conditions and/or disabilities, is a major national concern in the United States [1]. Regular physical activity, defined as 150 minutes of moderate physical activity per week [2], supports improved health and decreases the risk of obesity and chronic disease for people of all ages and abilities. Physical exercise also has important benefits for individuals with chronic health conditions such as arthritis [3]; depression [4, 5]; stroke [6]; lower-limb disabilities [7]; fibromyalgia [8, 9]; cardiopulmonary difficulties [10, 11]; multiple sclerosis [12]; Parkinson's disease [13]; and vestibular disorder [14]. In addition to physical benefits, engagement in physical activity provides psychological benefits for these individuals [15, 16]. Despite this evidence, less than half of all adults get the recommended amount of physical activity on a regular basis [17]. This issue becomes extremely serious during Coronavirus (COVID-19) pandemic [18]. The associated economic impact of physical inactivity is significant: annual health-care expenses are estimated at $860 billion for community-dwelling adults 50 years or older [2] with still additional workforce impacts [19]. These impacts are compounded by the fact that 80 percent of chronic conditions can be prevented or managed with regular physical activity [2]. Therefore, there is an urgent need to develop practical innovative exercise methods that *engage* individuals at all ages, including those with chronic health condition(s) and/or disability, *increase regular physical activity* levels, and *translate to improved health* with optimal functional ability and participation.

As noted above, typical physical activities may not always be feasible for individuals who suffer from disabilities or diseases, and may increase the risk of new and exacerbated chronic health conditions, compounded by advanced age. There is a critical need to tailor physical activity to an individual, based on their underlying capability, health risks, and movement goals. For example, different individuals may wish to strengthen different muscle groups, or have specific movement goals directed by a physical or occupational therapist.

In order to achieve those goals, we propose a **V**ersatile, **I**ndividualized, and **G**enerative **OR**chestrator (**VIGOR**) to motivate the movement of people (particularly those with limited mobility) [20]. To *Help*, *Push*, and *Coach* (**HPC**) users with various chronic health conditions to participate in restorative physical activities in the most effective way, the VIGOR system is designed to adapt to ensure an individualized experience that accounts for the personal, environmental, and social/cultural characteristics of the user [21]. **Figure 1** compares VIGOR with its competitors. The proposed VIGOR is unique in that it can provide a fully *personalized* user experience. Software products in the industry using virtual technology to encourage engagement in physical activity [23–25] include SaeboVR (www.saebo.com/saebovr), Nintendo Wii, and Verapy Therapy VAST (vast.rehab). Similar software products in Academia include OpenSim (opensim.stanford.edu) and QuaterNet (Facebook AI Research). Unlike those products, VIGOR integrates Tai-Chi, the traditional mind–body wellness and healing art [26, 27], with a series of data-driven computing technologies that will provide *customized* restorative physical activities for individuals with a broad range of chronic conditions and functional abilities. Our premise is that a user-friendly movement HPC system that may be conveniently utilized in sitting or standing positions, will empower individuals to increase their regular physical activity levels, and thus, improve health, functional ability, and participation in activities of everyday life. In this way, VIGOR emerges as an

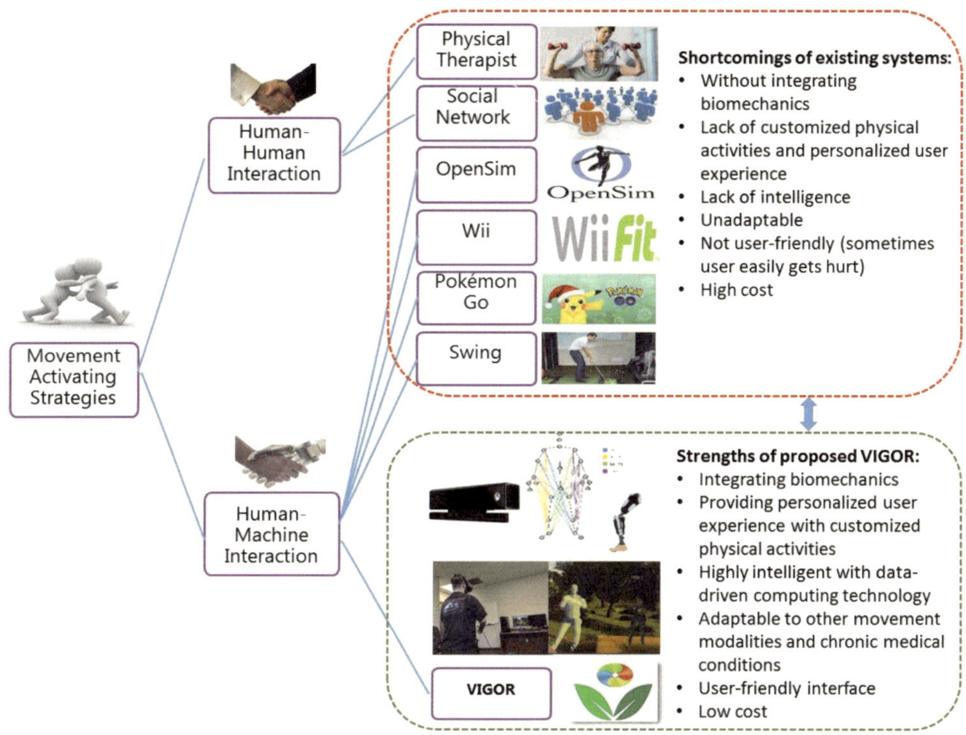

Figure 1.
Motivation and rationale for the proposed VIGOR system: a comparison between existing systems and VIGOR (online video [22]).

innovative, individualized and generative fitness modality that demonstrates connection of data, systems, and people for potential clinical benefits [20, 28].

In this research, we propose developing VIGOR within the context of Tai-Chi, a traditional mind–body wellness and healing art [26–28]. While our methods and framework can be applied to multiple exercise approaches, Tai-Chi is ideally suited to people with limited mobility, such as aging population and disabled people. Tai-Chi has documented benefits in improving balance as well as muscle strength, coordination, and endurance in multiple populations [26]. In addition, the low-impact nature of Tai-Chi is ideal for elderly individuals or groups with neuromusculoskeletal impairments. This exercise has low risks for musculoskeletal injury and joint damage while providing the many benefits of exercise.

While Tai-Chi is proven to have many health benefits, the underlying biomechanics of different choreography tailored to individual patient capabilities are difficult to identify. Knowing the "right" strategy for an individual from a kinematic trajectory alone is difficult without understanding underlying physiology. Biomechanical models can be used to determine the kinetics resulting in a desired kinematic trajectory [29–32], and then to coach the patient to activate the correct muscles to work toward their movement goals. Joint kinetics are more directly mapped to underlying muscular strength and capability compared to joint kinematics [32]. Thus, the incorporation of underlying biomechanics is critical for personalization of training sessions and mobility targets.

1.2 Rationale for the VIGOR system to address aging and chronic disability

Tai-Chi is characterized by low impact, flowing, and circular movements [13, 27]. The practice of these movements requires coordination and synchronization of a calm yet alert mind and a relaxed body [15, 16, 21]. It has enormous potential for improving physical and psychological functionality for users in both clinical and non-clinical settings by allowing flowing movements that offer body and mind benefits to users [28, 33, 34].

Enabled by deep learning technology, the proposed Tai-Chi based VIGOR offers several unique advantages as an individualized, effective, sustainable, and restorative fitness modality for users with movement-based chronic health conditions. The integration of Tai-Chi with four-dimensional (4D: the sensory data includes X-Y-Z plus a somatosensory signal [35, 36]) virtual-reality technology is both innovative and feasible in that: (1) Complex human movement can be deconstructed into primitive components/modes and deep learning methods [37] can be employed to accurately formulate the spatially and temporally dependent kinetic behavior as well as reconstruct incomplete joint movement or distorted movement caused by chronic health condition(s) [38]; (2) 4D kinetic behavior can be captured and reconstructed through modern sensors, actuators, and VR/AR technologies to generate seamless human-machine interaction; (3) Despite having significant storage and computation complexity, real-time kinetic analytics is applicable over a cutting-edge big-data engine and high-performance computing platform.

1.3 VIGOR's infrastructure

VIGOR aims to enable users an intelligent, four-dimensional (4D), partial control (e.g., virtual limb, which indicates that VIGOR can be driven by part of the inputs. In other words, VIGOR can tolerate and compensate for missing input when part of an input channel(s) is disabled), virtual-reality, and active-orthosis-enabled generative modality.

Figure 2 shows the infrastructure of the VIGOR system. A deep-learning-based virtual coach, which is trained by Tai-Chi master's kinetic data, is the core module of VIGOR. By applying experience (obtained via deep learning) with other related knowledge such as biomechanics and medical pathology, VIGOR measures a user's movements, evaluates his/her performance in comparison to the Tai-Chi master, and offers real-time visual and tactile feedback to the user. Far more than an on-site real-time Tai-Chi instructor, VIGOR also adapts the master movements to accommodate a wide range of mobility restrictions and improvements over time.

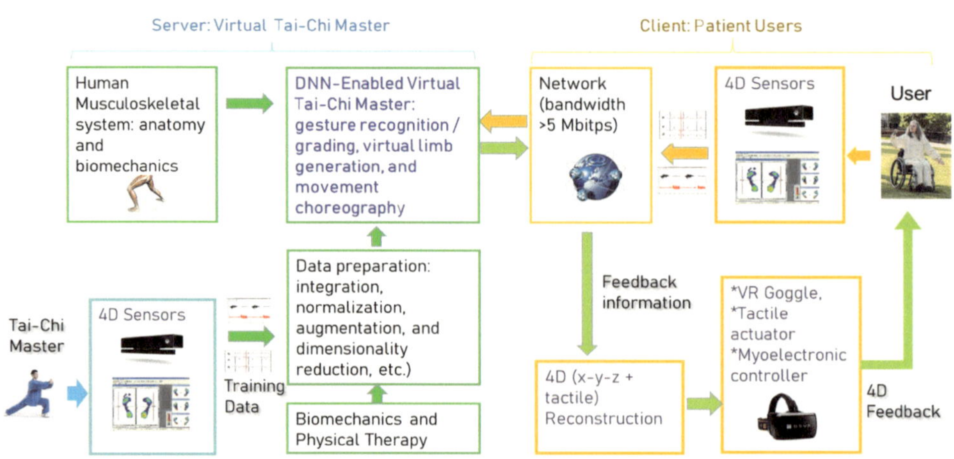

Figure 2.
Infrastructure of VIGOR.

The kinetic data for the Tai-Chi master and users are captured by different sensors, such as Microsoft Kinect and somatosensory sensors [39]. The fusion, transmission, storage, retrieval, management, and analytics [40] of sensory data are computationally and storage intensive. In VIGOR, an edge-computing-enabled network is exploited to connect the user with the virtual coach server. An edge server is employed to store and process the large volume of sensory data in real-time [41]. Integrated with Tensorflow, a deep learning library, VIGOR measures and predicts kinetic behavior of VIGOR users.

The system also provides the user with a multi-fold and panoramic 4D experience that includes visual, somatosensory information and direct physical support. 3D reconstruction and visualization with Unity3D allows the user to place themselves in a variety of different simulated spaces with a personalized virtual Tai-Chi coach walking them through Tai-Chi motions in a 3D world, supported by a soft-actuator based wearable device.

VIGOR is developed following "5S criteria" as follows: (1) Substantiation (or personalization) - VIGOR can provide user with personalized service according to their health condition and clinical requirements; (2) Simplicity - even those who are untrained or uneducated users can freely use VIGOR; (3) Skimpiness - only commodity hardware and software are used in VIGOR so that majority of people can afford it; (4) Scalability - VIGOR can satisfy the requirement of increasing number of users; (5) Speed - real-time response is needed to satisfy the requirement of users.

1.4 Research objectives and function modules of VIGOR

The major **objective** of the VIGOR is to develop a state-of-art deep learning system to help, push, and coach the people, particularly those suffering from mobile disability, so that they can get engaged in physical activities.

- *For the people who are not able to move* due to aging, disability or health issues, a **Helper** is needed to support their movement, virtually or physically. This is a network completion problem, which infers missing vertices (dysfunctional joints) and edges (i.e., dysfunctional muscles/bones). Section 4 will talk about the solution to this problem.

- *For the people who are reluctant to move*, a **Pusher** is needed to stimulate them through specific external audio/video/tactile stimulus (e.g., VR/AR, actuator). The reconstruction of physics stimulus will be addressed in Subsection 2.2.

- *For the people who do not know how to move*, a **Coach** is needed to recognize/score their' motion and send them real-time feedback/instruction (Subsections 3.2 and 3.3); or design individualized and optimized exercise according to their health condition or medical requirement. These two problems are motion recognition (Section 3) and generation (Section 5), respectively.

As a matter of fact, machine learning approaches ignore the fundamental biomechanics law and clinical regulations for human motion and thus may result in ill-posed problems. Additionally, deeper and wider deep neural networks (DNNs) often require large sets of labeled data for effective training and suffer from extremely high computational complexity, preventing them from being deployed in real-time systems. As a result, there is a need to incorporate domain knowledge into DNNs [42, 43]. As one of the major contributions of this project, domain knowledge will be infused into DNNs through data augmentation, customizing loss function, or embedding knowledge block into NN as an independent module (e.g., dynamics-guided discriminator in the motion choreography module).

Enabled by the deep neural network and multimodal human-machine-interaction techniques, the VIGOR system consists of the following function modules:

- *Real-time 4D human-machine interaction based on robust data acquisition, transmission, and re-construction methods* (Section 2). It is challenging to integrate, represent and analyze heterogeneous 4D temporal data in proper data formats, which is applicable over various affordable hardware instruments. In this task, a proper uniform data format characterizing the human kinetics across heterogeneous hardware platforms is studied. In addition, to facilitate the interaction between user and VIGOR, two-way communications are investigated.

- *Identification of a user's kinetic movement* (Section 3). To help, push and coach (HPC) users (including people with mobile disability) in real time, VIGOR needs to identify a user's kinetic behavior and respond users with prompt instructions. Major research challenges are (1) the normalization of the kinetics of users (including the people with limited mobility), (2) the formulation Tai-Chi movement philosophy using neural network, and (3) the metrics about movement grading. The technical contributions of VIGOR include: (1) normalizing sensory data spatially, temporally, and kinetically, and removing occlusion using spherical interpolation and Kalman filtering algorithms; (2) deriving reference Tai-Chi kinetic patterns of using temporal neural network such as long-short term memory (LSTM); (3) grading users' kinetic behavior using entropy; and (4) enriching kinetic data using inverse dynamics theory.

- *Adaptive virtual limb generation* (Section 4). To motivate a user who has had a limb amputated to move, VIGOR provides the user with a pleasurable sensation experience that the limb is still there by generating a virtual limb. To this end, a major challenge is the difficulty in generating the adaptive motion of the virtual limb based on the observed kinetic behaviors of functional body parts. In this task, deep neural network regression is designed for real-time virtual limb generation and then time series prediction model [44] is used to improve the consistency of generated kinetics sequence. A hierarchical visible autoencoder is developed and evaluated for the adaptive virtual limb generation according to the kinetic behavior of functional body-parts, which are measured by heterogeneous kinetic sensors. The virtual limbs can be reconstructed on VR/AR platform and active orthoses [45].

- *Creating individualized movement choreography* (Section 5). A unique feature of VIGOR is its ability to create customized movement choreography for individual users based on their observed health conditions. One of the most challenging issues in deep learning enabled choreography is how to balance the training reliability and the creativity of neural network. In consideration of complex body action coordination in human motion, visible deep neural networks integrating biomechanics and DNNs are developed to generate Tai-Chi choreography. Specifically, knowledge-guided neural network architectures of LSTM, generative adversarial networks (GAN) [46], and their combinations with multiple data modality are designed to create customized movement choreography for individual users based on their health conditions and clinical rehabilitation requirements. New training methods based on the polynomial-based Hessian-free Newton–Raphson optimizer [47] is also created.

Each research objective along with the specific challenges and tasks will be described in more detail in Sections 2–5 individually.

2. Real-time 4D human-machine interaction

The challenge of Objective 1 is to provide real-time (prompt HPC feedback) and scalable (to support multiple-user) human-machine interaction environment based on affordable hardware instruments with heterogeneous modality. To address the challenge, real-time 4D data acquisition and two-way communication are investigated.

2.1 Acquisition of 4D sensory data

Figure 3 shows the basic input and output equipment of VIGOR. A Microsoft Kinect and a foot pressure sensor are used as input equipment to acquire kinetic data (or 4D sensory data) of an VIGOR user. Virtual reality goggles, such as the Oculus Rift or HTC Vive, tactile actuators, and active orthoses are used as output equipment that work together to depict 4D feedback to the user.

2.1.1 Acquisition and processing of kinematic data

The Microsoft Kinect collects the kinematic data of the Tai-Chi master (for training purposes) and the user. Through Kinect, we can obtain joints' transient position $\langle x, y, z \rangle_t^k$ and corresponding Quaternion rotation [48] $\left\langle \cos\left(\frac{\theta}{2}\right), \sin\left(\frac{\theta}{2}\right)\vec{v} \right\rangle^k$, where θ is an angle around unit axis $\vec{v}$, t is the time, and k is the joint identifier. Quaternions [48] are considered to represent the rotation of a rigid body in 3D space using four degrees-of-freedom (DOFs).

Quaternions are superior to many other traditional rotation formulation methods because they completely avoid gimbal-lock [49]. In VIGOR, Quaternions are used in 4D reconstruction over Unity3D platform and acquisition of kinetic signal. On the other hand, as a Quaternion is specified with reference to an arbitrary axis vector it is not a good choice in rotation recognition. In VIGOR, Euler angles $\langle \alpha, \beta, \gamma \rangle$, which represent the angles rotating around axis Z, X, Y respectively (denoted as $\langle yaw, pitch, roll \rangle$ in some literature) are adopted in gesture recognition.

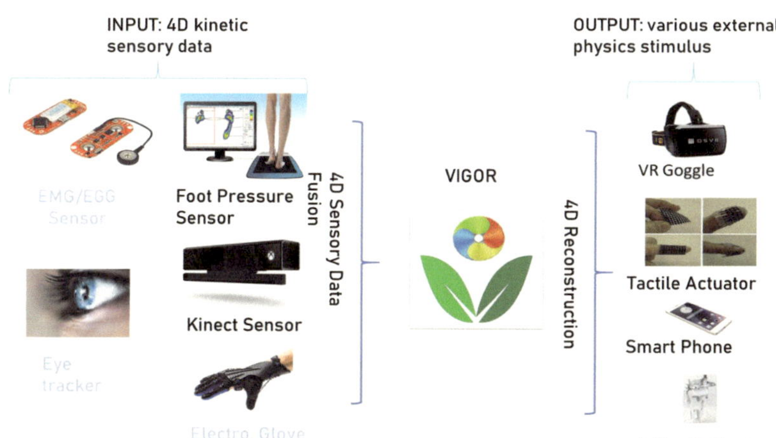

Figure 3.
Input&output instruments (the optional hardware is highlighted in light color).

VIGOR stores the captured kinetic data in JavaScript Object Notation (JSON) format, which includes joint position $\left(\langle x, y, z\rangle_t^k\right)$, quaternion rotation $\left(\left\langle \cos\left(\frac{\theta}{2}\right), \sin\left(\frac{\theta}{2}\right)\vec{v} \right\rangle_t^k\right)$, tracking status (0: invisible; 1: referred; 2: observable), and potentially forces $\left(\mathbf{f}_t^k\right)$ and moments, etc. Tracking status indicates whether or not the joint is observable by the sensor. The forces and moments are derived by inverse dynamics analysis.

Due to measurement error or unavoidable occlusion, a joint is not always observable or tractable by the kinetic sensor. Spherical linear intERPolation (SLERP) [50] and Kalman filtering techniques (be discussed in Section 3.1) are employed to compensate the missing data. As illustrated in our preliminary online video [22], SLERP can effectively address those short-term missed-tracking joints (namely tracking status = 0 or 1).

2.1.2 Acquisition of tactile data

Besides Kinect, other acquisition instruments such as accelerometers, orientation sensors, and strain gauges [39] are also considered for the VIGOR system. As indicated above, a foot pressure sensor is used to obtain the ground reaction force F_t for inverse dynamic analysis. Furthermore, electromyography (EMG) [39] is selectively employed to evaluate and record the electrical activity produced by skeletal muscles. The EMG signal is characterized by a frequency range of several hertz to over 1 kHz and by amplitudes ranging from fractions of a microvolt to a few thousand microvolts. Electromyographic signals can be analyzed to detect activation level or to analyze the biomechanics of users' movement. To acquire high-quality EMG signals from localized muscle region, identification of localized muscle region of users, noise reduction and grounding practices (to eliminate extraneous electrical noise), electrode site preparation and placement (to minimize the detection of irrelevant bioelectrical signals) and appropriate differential signal preamplification and preliminary signal conditioning (to further enhance signal-to-noise ratio) can be conducted. EMG signals can be classified to detect movements of limb. Our active/powered orthosis system, which enables users for movement, has EMG and Internal measurement Unit (IMU) sensors. Those sensors can monitor body movement and muscle activity and send the measurement data to the server.

2.2 Reconstruction of 4D data

4D kinetic feedback/instruction is reconstructed through virtual reality, tactile actuators, and motoring system that drives the active orthosis. (1) *VR/AR facility*, which can visualize the kinetics of human body in Quaternion format [48, 49] (acceptable by Unity3D VR/AR SDK). (2) *Tactile actuators*, through which VIGOR can directly guide users with somatosensory feedback. Tactile actuators potentially used in VIGOR include Eccentric Rotating Mass (ERM), Linear Resonant Actuator (LRA), Piezo, and Electro-Active polymers (EAP) with high fidelity of sensations, and excellent durability. (3) *Active orthosis* [51], which enables users with direct physical support through functional electrical stimulation (F.E.S) [51] or robotic exoskeletons [45].

2.3 Developing communication and edge-computing protocols

2.3.1 Real-time, two-way communication

Two-way communications are of key importance in the proposed system, since the information needs to be exchanged in a real-time manner. The challenges of the communication protocol for the proposed VIGOR include: (1) Real-time communication: Information in the VIGOR system needs to be conveyed in real time. If there is a significant delay in the communications, synchronization between the Tai-Chi master and user will be lost and the user will experience a disturbed rhythm. (2) High communication throughput: When there are many users, all the corresponding multimodal sensory data and feedback information need to be conveyed in the network, thus incurring a substantial requirement for communication bandwidth. (3) Two-way communications: The communications are between the virtual Tai-Chi master and users with mutual interactions. Therefore, it could be sub-optimal if one-way communications are considered separately. (4) Dynamics awareness: The communications may be optimized together with the physical dynamics of the virtual Tai-Chi master and users (namely the motions).

To address the above challenges, first, VIGOR can be modeled as a cyber physical system (CPS) [52, 53] and then the bandwidth can be analyzed for controlling the physical dynamics. Last, the detailed communication protocol can be designed and evaluated with the whole system.

2.3.2 Deployment of VIGOR on affordable hardware using edge computing

Edge computing enables real-time knowledge generation and application to occur at the source of the data close to user device [54, 55], which makes it particularly suitable for the proposed latency-sensitive system. An edge server can be adapted to serve multiple users through interaction with their devices. There are communication and computing trade-offs between the edge server and each user device. Data could either be locally processed at the user device or else be transmitted to and processed at the edge server. Different strategies introduce different communication costs, resulting in different delay performance. To provide the best quality of experience for users, the following tasks are involved: (1) Identification and modularization of computing tasks: the computing tasks of data preprocessing, kinetic movement recognition, and individualization of movement choreography need to be identified and the corresponding computing overheads (CPU cycles, memory) need to be determined. (2) Design, prototyping and enhancement of offloading schemes: Based on the results of bandwidth and delay analysis as well as delay performance requirement, computation offloading schemes need to be developed to determine which computing tasks should be performed locally at the user device and which computation tasks should be offloaded to the edge server. As shown in **Figure 4**, an illustrative concept demonstration about edge-computing-enabled VIGOR is given in our online video [56].

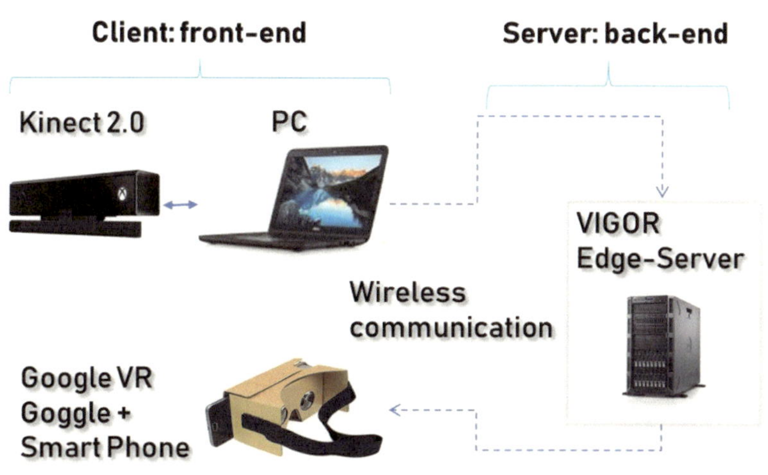

Figure 4.
Edge-computing-enabled VIGOR deployed on commodity hardware (demo in online video [56]).

3. Identification and scoring of user's kinetic movement

To help, push and coach (HPC) users with movement disabilities in real time, VIGOR is featured with: (1) an enriched dataset by introducing kinetic data (specified by time series [57–59]), which is derived from the measured kinematic data, into the neural network; (2) compensating with any missing kinetic data introduced by users' disability. Identification of a user's kinetic behavior during movement mainly involves the following research tasks:

3.1 Preprocessing pipeline for kinetic movement identification

Data preprocessing operations play an indispensable role in VIGOR because:

- *Input data is of a heterogeneous nature*. For example, different users have variable sizes; sensors may have various viewing angles; users may not always be located in a deterministic position; and the two time-series data sets may not be synchronized. As a result, scaling, rotating, translating, and dynamic time warping (DTW) are needed to normalize the original input data.

- *The input data set may be incomplete*. For example, occlusion inevitably leads to missing data; Musculoskeletal forces and moments exerted over the joints from muscles cannot be directly obtained from the sensors [60]; some input channels are not enabled (e.g., partial control) for users with mobility-based chronic conditions (i.e., partial control). In the implementation of VIGOR, Kalman filtering, inverse dynamics, and time-series prediction are employed to handle the incomplete data [35, 61].

- *The measurement-induced noise is significant*.

Figure 5 shows the flowchart of data preprocessing of VIGOR [36, 41, 62, 63]. $\left(\theta, \vec{v}\right)$, where θ is the rotation angle about axis $\vec{v}$, indicates a joint's Quaternion rotation; $\langle x, y, z\rangle$ denotes a joint's position; f_t indicates a joint's applied force, which is derived from inverse dynamics; $\langle \alpha, \beta, \gamma\rangle$ indicates a joint's rotation under normalized Joint Coordinate System (JCS) – Euler angle. Its main implementation techniques include data fusion, inverse dynamics analysis, spatial normalization, Kalman filtering, and reconstruction of disable input channels. The kinetic data is stored in JSON format.

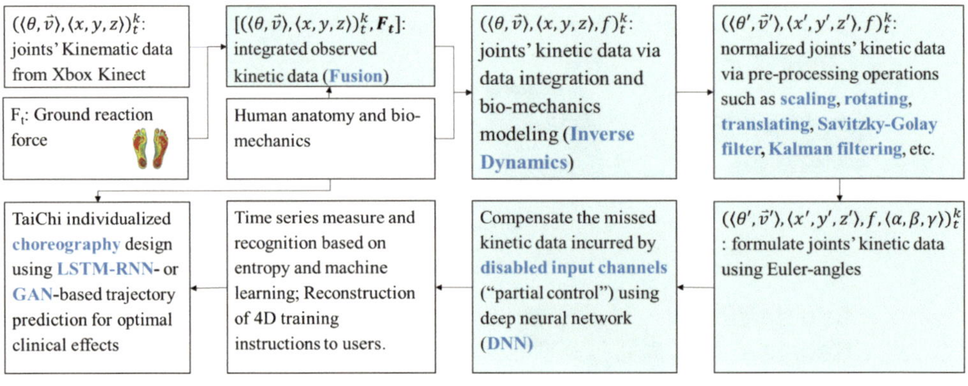

Figure 5.
Flowchart of VIGOR's Preprocessing for kinetic movement identification.

3.1.1 Formulating musculoskeletal kinetic features

Inverse dynamics analysis (IDA), which is derived from Newton-Euler Equations [60, 64–68], aims to calculate unknown kinetic information (the net joint forces and moments) from measured kinematic information (e.g., position, velocities and accelerations of joints) and measured kinetic information (e.g., ground reaction forces). As illustrated in **Figure 5**, given joint locations $\langle x_i, y_i, z_i \rangle$, Euler rotation $\langle \alpha_i, \beta_i, \gamma_i \rangle$ where i denotes the identity of a joint, and ground-reaction force F, the joint force f_i and other musculoskeletal kinetic features can be computed via IDA.

As illustrated in **Figure 5**, VIGOR employs *inverse dynamics* to compute internal joint forces and moments with given ground reaction forces. Inverse dynamics is implemented by dividing the human body into multiple connected rigid bodies [69, 70], which correspond to relevant anatomical segments such as the thigh, calf, foot, arm, etc. The model's anthropometric properties (e.g., the mass and moment of inertia) are derived from statistical analysis. In addition, it is assumed that each joint is rotationally frictionless. The proposed methods in **Figure 5** can be customized to investigate the biomechanical response of human motion by considering different health issues such as cerebral palsy, poliomyelitis, spinal cord injury, and muscular dystrophy [67].

3.1.2 Spatial normalization

As addressed in Section 2, we can acquire joint positions and rotations, which are denoted as $\langle x, y, z \rangle$ and $\left\langle \theta, \vec{v} \right\rangle$ respectively. Both need to be normalized to ease and boost the gesture recognition: (1) *Normalization of Joint Rotations* through the interchangeable conversion among quaternion $\left\langle \theta, \vec{v} \right\rangle$, Euler angle α, β, γ, and joint positions $\langle x, y, z \rangle$ [71]. (2) *Normalization of Joint Positions* using bone scaling [61], axis-oriented rotating of view angle, origin translating (which makes a user positioned at the center of a sensor), re-constructing $\langle x, y, z \rangle$ according to joint rotation [49], and polishing the kinetic curve using a Savitzky–Golay filter. Our preliminary experimental results demonstrate that the normalization techniques addressed above can greatly improve the quality of data (less noise and smoother kinetic performance) so as to achieve higher recognition [36, 41, 61].

3.1.3 Recovering occlusion-induced missing data

During sensory data acquisition, unavoidable occlusion may introduce missing data or lost-tracking. VIGOR employs spherical linear interpolation (SLERP) to fix the issues caused by short-term occlusion [35], and employs Kalman filter [72–74] to fix the missing information (including both position and rotation) caused by long-term occlusion. A preliminary comparison between the raw and preprocessed physical rehabilitation kinematic data is available on our online video [62, 63].

3.1.4 Normalization of the kinetics of users with limited mobility

In order to recognize the kinetic movement of users with disabilities, VIGOR normalizes their kinetic data by compensating the missing data incurred by disabled input channels: in the event that several input channels are disabled, the VIGOR model is able to construct the void input channels by taking the advantage of correlation among all inputs. Compensation can normalize the input data so that

VIGOR can achieve higher recognition rate, and its psychological and physiological benefits to users are also under our investigation. **Figure 6** demonstrates the application of deep neural network [37, 75] on compensating the missing channels introduced by limited mobility. As our preliminary contribution, multilayer perceptron (MLP), temporal convolutional neural network (tCNN) [46], and autoencoder methods are employed to construct disabled legs and the resulted recognition accuracy is improved [20].

3.2 Entropy-oriented scoring of human motion

The proposed research employs entropy [76] to grade a user's movement behavior, which is defined as a times series of joint kinetic features such as positions and rotations. The distance/dissimilarity between two time series can be measured in time-domain or frequency-domain [58, 59]. In time-domain, Approximate Entropy (AppEn) and Sample Entropy (SampEn) [76, 77] can be employed to formulate the regularity and predictability about the normalized Euclidean distance between the time-series of users' and reference data.

As our preliminary work, **Figure 7** compares the entropy values of an advanced Tai-Chi user and a beginner. The whole Tai-Chi set is divided into multiple subsequence (or clip), which consists of 25 to 100 frames, and the comparison is made clip-by-clip. In **Figure 7**, each subsequence consists of 25 frames. It is observed that an advanced Tai-Chi user has smaller entropy than a beginner. Besides the overall entropy of a user, VIGOR also provides the entropy of each joint so that the virtual Tai-Chi coach can provide accurate instruction to users.

Entropy or cross-entropy analysis can be performed for the time-series in the frequency domain which is derived from discrete Fourier transformation (DFT) or discrete wavelet transformation (DWT) [58, 59]. A hybrid metric that combines both time-domain and frequency-domain information may be considered as well.

3.3 Human motion identification based on machine learning

Many model construction techniques have been developed for time series recognition [59, 78, 79], including K-Nearest-Neighbor (KNN) [80], Support Vector Machines (SVMs) [81, 82], neural networks, decision trees [83, 84], Bayesian networks, the Hidden Markov model (HMM), LSTM-RNN, etc.

In this work, the recognition accuracy of the aforementioned classifiers with respect to three benchmark datasets was determined: *Dataset I: UTD Multimodal Human Action Dataset* (UTD MHAD [85]), *Dataset II: UTKinect-Action3D* [86], and

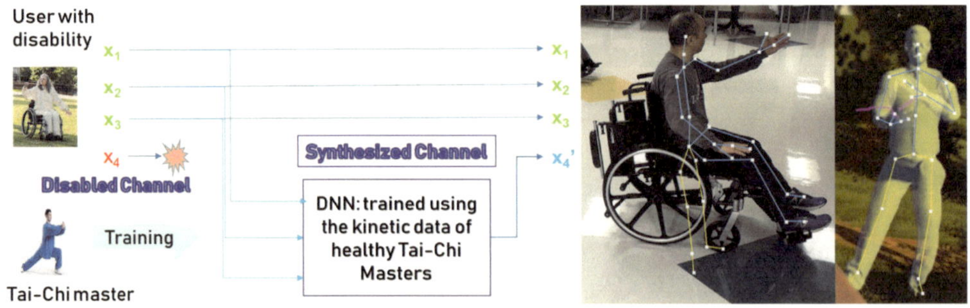

Figure 6.
Normalizing the kinetics of user with limited mobility: (a) Compensation of disabled input channels via Deep Neural Network; (b) tCNN-enabled compensated kinetic status of a wheel-chaired user, who receives "virtual functional legs" (in yellow color).

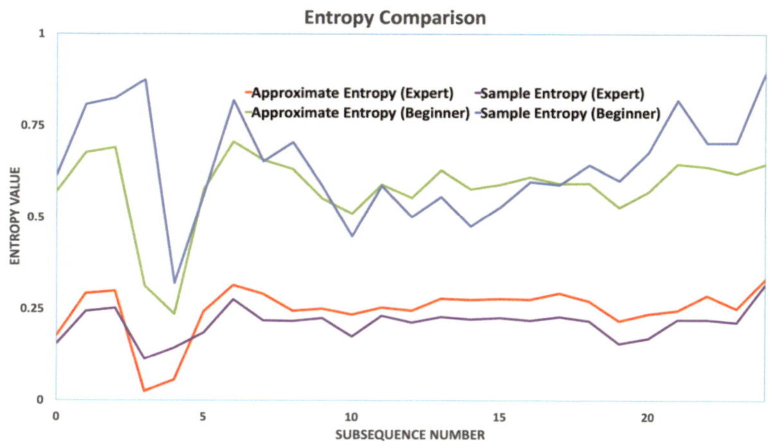

Figure 7.
AppEn and SampEn for 25 joints: Comparison of an advanced users and beginner (Each subsequence consists of 25 frames): beginner has larger entropy.

Dataset III: Tai-Chi Yang-Style 24 movement [22, 41] (an in-house Kinect skeletal dataset collected for Tai-Chi training). The experimental results showed that SVM and LSTM-RNN surpasses the other classifiers; particularly, LSTM-RNN has a superior recognition accuracy in case of limited number of training data (e.g., 200 training samples). However, LSTM-RNN suffers from unsatisfactory time performance [35]. Scalable algorithms for temporal neural network such as LSTM-RNN and temporal convolutional network (tCNN) need to be developed [46].

In this work, a musculoskeletal biomechanics guided loss function is used to formulate the objective of kinetics classifier:

$$\mathcal{L}(\theta) = L\big(f(\mathbf{X},\theta),\mathbf{y}\big) + \varrho\mathcal{R}(\theta), \tag{1}$$

where $\mathbf{y}$ is the pre-determined movement identity; $f(\mathbf{X}, \theta)$ is predicting movement identity of kinetics sequence $\mathbf{X} = \left\{(\langle\langle x_t^k, y_t^k, z_t^k\rangle, \mathbf{f})_t^k\rangle\right\}_{t=t_0}^{t_m}$ (as defined in **Figure 5**, t is time step ranging from t_0 through t_m, k is joint's identity); $\theta \in \mathfrak{R}^n$ indicates the parameters (weight and bias) of neural network; $\mathcal{R}(\theta) : \mathfrak{R}^n \rightarrow \mathfrak{R}$ is the regularizer, whose importance is controlled by regularization strength $\varrho \in \mathfrak{R}$; and $\mathcal{L}(\theta) : \mathfrak{R}^n \rightarrow \mathfrak{R}$ is actually regularized loss. The corresponding optimization method is called batch optimizer.

3.4 Reconstruction of 4D instruction/feedback for users

VIGOR can be also regarded as a real-time coaching system to help users improve their physical rehabilitation movement for optimal clinical effect. According to the measure and recognition result discussed above, VTCS generates real-time 4D instructions or guidance to users over virtual reality or augmented reality (AR) platform, as shown in the online video [22, 87, 88] addressed in our preliminary work.

4. Adaptive virtual limb generation

To relieve the physical and psychological suffering of people with limited mobility, VIGOR develops an adaptive (versatile to various types of disability) and full-body-driven virtual limb generation system (all measurable body-parts will be used to formulate virtual limbs). The related technical contributions include: (1) According to specified kinetic script (e.g., dancing, running, etc.) and users' physical conditions, a hierarchical network is extracted from human musculoskeletal network, which is fabricated by multiple body components (e.g., muscles, bones, and joints, etc.) that are biomechanically, functionally, or neurally correlated with each other and exhibit mostly non-divergent kinetic behaviors. (2) The generated limb can be reconstructed over the VR/AR system, tactile actuator system, and motoring system.

4.1 Pipeline of adaptive virtual limb generation

The proposed work employs deep learning techniques such as autoencoder to generate virtual limbs [89] according to the observed kinetic behaviors of other body parts based on the following hypothesis: (1) The human body consists of multiple components such as muscles, bones, and joints, which are correlated with each other mechanically, neurally, and/or functionally. (2) Deep learning techniques such as autoencoder can be used to capture the kinetic pattern of human movement.

Figure 8(a) shows the flowchart of the adaptive virtual limb generation, which consists of the following critical aspects: (1) Formulating human musculoskeletal network [91] according to the functional, mechanical and neural correlation between each body component (muscle, joint, or bone). (2) Deriving hierarchical network (in the configuration of forest data structure) from the human musculoskeletal network according to the physical status of users, where the virtual limbs will form the leaves of a hierarchical tree. (3) Building visible autoencoder neural network according to the hierarchical network so that the kinetic behavior can be constructed according to the kinetic behavior of user's functional body parts measured by heterogeneous sensors. (4) Training the addressed visible autoencoder neural network according to specific human movement script such as walking, jogging, dancing, or any other physical activity. (5) Representing kinematic behavior about virtual limbs using VR/AR, tactile actuators, and active orthoses, which can directly stimulate users. **Figure 8(b)** shows the screenshot of virtual limb generation.

4.2 Multivariate time series-based kinetics generation of Virtual Limbs

Adaptive and full-body-driven virtual limb generation can (1) engage various individuals with limited mobility in regular physical activities, (2) accelerate the rehabilitation of patients, and (3) release users' phantom limb pain.

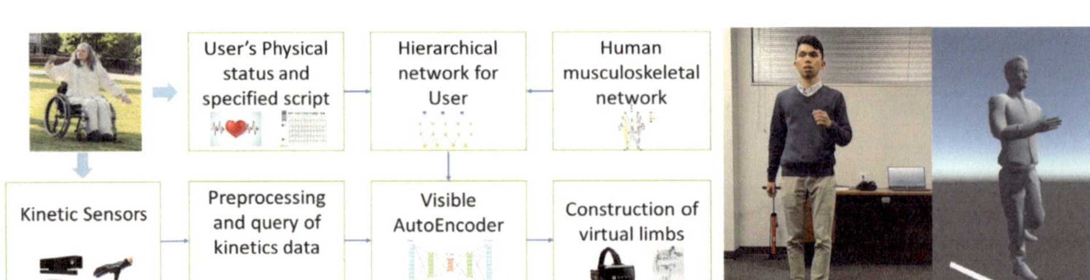

Figure 8.
(a) The flowchart of the proposed adaptive virtual limb generation based on multi-correlation hierarchical autoencoder; (b) Snapshot of virtual limb generation – walking by moving arms (online video [90]).

Virtual limb generation is a generative time series problem. **Figure 9** shows the pipeline of kinetics generation (a multivariate time-series) and correction of kinetic sequence of the virtual limbs.

- $\mathbf{Y}_t^{measured} = \{(\langle\langle x_t^i, y_t^i, z_t^i\rangle, \mathbf{f})_t^i\rangle\}_{t=t_0}^{t_m}$ denotes the measured kinetic sequence of functional body parts. As defined in **Figure 5**, t is time step ranging from t_0 through t_m, k is the identity of joints that are related to function body parts.

- $\mathbf{Y}_t^{virtual} = \{\left(\left\langle\left\langle x_t^j, y_t^j, z_t^j\right\rangle, \mathbf{f}\right)_t^j\right\rangle\}_{t=t_0}^{t_m}$ denotes the generated kinetic sequence of virtual limbs, t is time step ranging from t_0 through t_m, j is the identity of joints that are related to virtual limbs.

As illustrated in **Figure 6**, we can generate the the kinetics of the wheel-chaired Tai-Chi practitioner according to the movement of his/her arms, which are functional and healthy. This work employs deep neural network to generate $\mathbf{Y}_t^{virtual}$ using $\mathbf{Y}_t^{measured}$:

$$\mathbf{Y}_t^{virtual} = f\left(\mathbf{Y}_t^{measured}, \theta\right) \tag{2}$$

where $f\left(\mathbf{Y}_t^{measured}, \theta\right)$ is the output of deep neural network.

4.2.1 Loss function for the Generation of virtual limbs' kinetics

In this work, a musculoskeletal biomechanics guided loss function is used to formulate the objective of generated virtual limbs' kinetics:

$$\mathcal{L}(\theta) = L\left(\mathbf{Y}^{virtual}, \mathbf{Y}\right) + \varrho\mathcal{R}(\theta) + L_{biomechanics}\left(\mathbf{Y}^{virtual}\right). \tag{3}$$

In Eq. (3), $(\mathbf{Y}^{virtual}, \mathbf{Y})$ indicates labelled training data; $\mathbf{Y}^{virtual}$ is the expected kinetic of virtual limbs; $\theta \in \mathfrak{R}^n$ indicates the parameters (weight and bias) of neural network; $\mathcal{R}(\theta) : \mathfrak{R}^n \to \mathfrak{R}$ is the regularizer, whose importance is controlled by regularization strength $\varrho \in \mathfrak{R}$; $L_{biomechanics}\left(\mathbf{Y}^{virtual}\right)$ denotes the bio-mechanics violation of generated kinetics with weigh $\gamma \in \mathfrak{R}$ and this work uses kinetic imbalance of human body to measure $L_{biomechanics}$; and $\mathcal{L}(\theta) : \mathfrak{R}^n \to \mathfrak{R}$ is actually regularized loss.

4.2.2 Correction of generated kinetics using time-series prediction model

The kinetic sequence of virtual limbs does not behave smoothly. This work corrects $\mathbf{Y}_t^{virtual}$ using Auto-Regressive Integrated Moving Average (ARIMA) [44] time-series prediction model. ARIMA model is fitted to time series data for pattern recognition and forecasting. The AR part of ARIMA indicates that the evolving variable of interest is regressed on its prior (or historical) values. The MA part

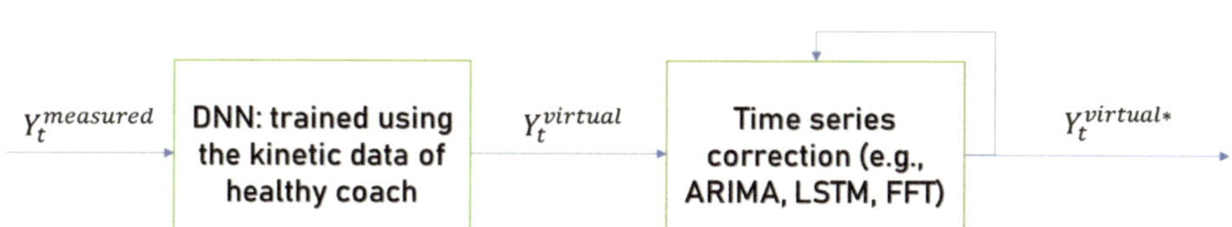

Figure 9.
Generation and correction of the kinetics of virtual limbs.

indicates that the regression error is actually a linear combination of error terms whose values occurred contemporaneously and at various times in the past. The I (for "integrated") indicates that the data values have been replaced with the difference between their values and the previous values. ARIMA is defined as:

$$\mathbf{Y}_t^{virtual*} = c + \sum_{k=1}^{p} \phi_k \mathbf{Y}_{t-k}^{virtual} + \sum_{k}^{q} \psi_k \varepsilon_{t-k} + \varepsilon_t \quad (4)$$

where $\mathbf{Y}_t^{virtual}$ is the differenced series (it may have been differenced more than once). The "predictors" on the right hand side include both lagged values of $\mathbf{Y}_t^{virtual}$ and lagged errors. Eq. (4) is also called ARIMA(p, d, q) model, where p is the order of the autoregressive part; d is the degree of first differencing involved; q is the order of the moving average part.

Any time series may be split into the following components: base Level, trend, seasonality and error. The coefficient of the ARIMA model is determined through autocorrelation [44] and the correlation of the series with its previous values.

4.3 Formulating the kinetics of virtual limbs using the measured kinetics of functional body parts

As described in Eqs. (2) and (4), the generation of virtual limb kinetics consists of two steps: (1) create preliminary kinetics of virtual limbs according to the measured kinetics of functional body parts; and (2) correct the preliminary kinetics using time series prediction models such as ARIMA. This subsection will focus on Step (1) because it faces more technical challenges.

4.3.1 Configuration of network architecture according human anatomy

It is known that any system can be regarded as a hierarchical structure (i.e., system → subsystem → sub-subsystem, …). As illustrated in **Figure 10(a)**, the human body system can be always divided into sub-components that are mechanically correlated. Inspired by the Bayesian network, we propose a visible and hierarchical neural network (VHNN), which is derived from human anatomy, to accurately formulate a system. As illustrated in **Figure 10(b)**, a sample visible and hierarchical neural network, which is directly derived from the human body

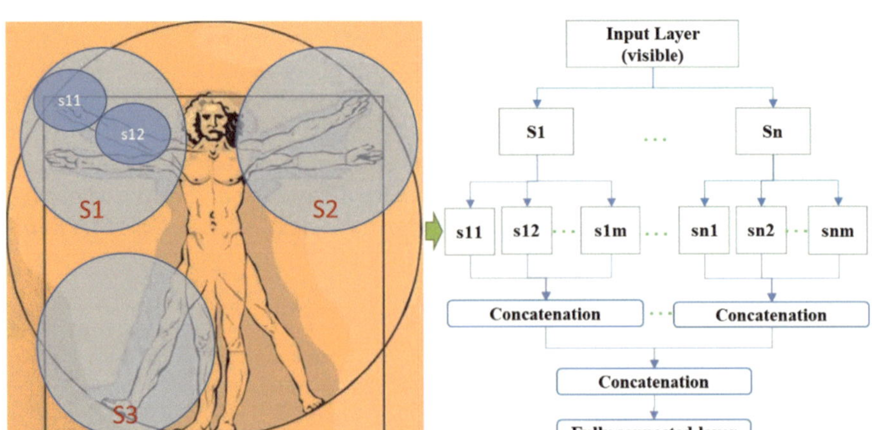

Figure 10.
(a) Hierarchical human anatomy; (b) visible and hierarchical neural network derived from human anatomy.

system, is employed to specify the musculoskeletal kinematics. The VHNN can be employed in virtual limb generation, 4D kinetic behavior recognition, and individualized Tai-Chi choreography (to be discussed in the remaining sections). Preliminary experimental results demonstrate that VHNN is superior to a classical neural network from the point of view of training speed and stability.

4.3.2 Example: generating virtual legs based on arm movement using VHNN

A neural network is trained to generate the kinetic status of hip, knees, and feet according to the kinetic status of shoulders, elbows, and arms captured by 4D sensors [90]. As illustrated in **Figure 11 (a)–(d)**, four network architectures are investigated in this research: (a) multiple layer perceptron (MLP); (b) denoising autoencoder (a classical autoencoder architecture); (c) visible and hierarchical neural network with two subsystems (VHNN2); and (c) VHNN with four subsystems (VHNN4). It can be observed that VHNN splits the input tensor and then feeds the split tensor into multiple smaller, parallelized autoencoders. Thus, data for each joint can be calculated in parallel with their own respective autoencoder. The aforementioned parallelized autoencoder pipelines are simplified stacked autoencoders, allowing for optimization of specific, key tasks rather than one large task. A video playlist of the generation of virtual legs based on VHNN may be found at [92].

As illustrated in **Figure 9**, the generated kinetics of virtual limbs can be corrected using time-series models such as ARIMA.

As illustrated in **Table 1**, the proposed VPNN architecture has proven to have overall superior results compared to previous work. Decreased training time compared to previous autoencoders architectures can be observed due to the parallelization of simpler autoencoders, increasing efficiency by easing optimization. This is done by allowing autoencoders to train on specific gestures in a whole movement. In addition, it does not exhibit data-hungry tendencies that state-of-the-art models exhibit, allowing it to be trained on small amounts of data.

Lower ground truth error can be seen in the VPNN-AE-2 versus VPNN-AE-4. This is due to training data having no anomalies that real-time data can exhibit. While VPNN-AE-2 with single-correlation works better when testing against ground truth data, VPNN-AE-4 with double-correlation works better in real-time as the patient may not follow the Tai-Chi movements correctly. This causes worse ground truth error as the added complexity of the architecture increases noise

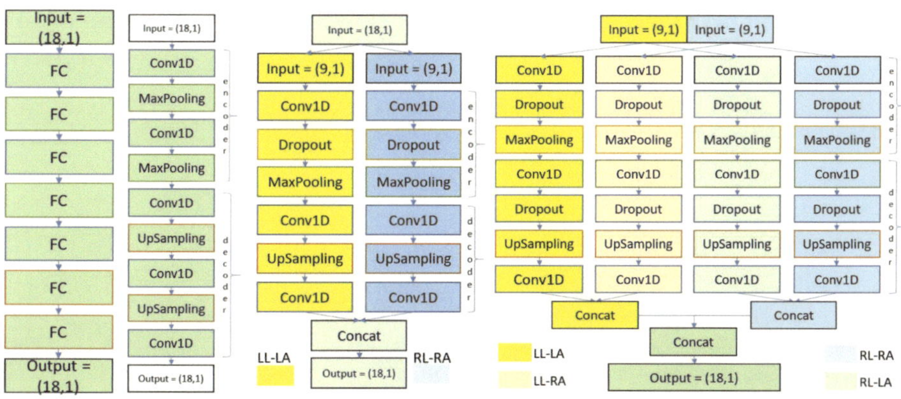

Figure 11.
Generation of virtual legs from moving arms using various architecture: (a) MLP; (b) denoising autoencoder (a classical architecture); (c) two thread (subsystem) visible and hierarchical autoencoder neural network (VHNN-AE-2); (d) four-thread VHNN (VHNN-AE-4) (notes: LL-LA indicates virtual left-leg induced by left-arm; LL-RA indicates virtual right-leg induced by right arm) (online video: [92]).

NN architecture	Training time per step	Training time for 1 K epochs	Convergence in epoch	Ground truth error	Online video
MLP	NA	NA	250	9515.51	[93]
Denoising Autoencoder	108 − 110 μs	9 m 15 s	1000	2107.46	[94]
VPNN-Autoencoder-2	30 − 31 μs	2 m 44 s	500	276.68	[95]
VPNN-Autoencoder-4	52 − 57 μs	4 m 37 s	800	366.15	[96]

Table 1.
Time-performance of virtual-legs generation using visible and hierarchical autoencoder neural network (VHNN), which is derived from human anatomy (Intel Core i9-7900X, 1x NVIDIA GTX1080 Ti, 64GB RAM; MLP does not employ GPU).

during output, but enables better patient-error tolerance. Because of this additional noise produced of VPNN-AE-4, improvements through larger training datasets, more sophisticated pre- and post-processing of data, as well as improved NN architecture could be achieved.

4.4 Construction of virtual limb using active orthosis

In order to provide users with physical support, the generated virtual limb can be re-constructed on motoring system to drive Hip–knee–ankle–foot orthoses (HKAFOs) [97, 98]. Paralysis of hip abductor muscles is one of the most common reasons for prescribing HKAFOs. They can incorporate flexion–extension and abduction–adduction control and have free or locking joints [99]. Different from passive and semi-active orthoses, the HKAFOs have basically built-in power supplies, one or more actuators for moving the joint, the sensors for getting feedback data [97].

The designed active orthosis is shown in **Figure 12(A)**. Knee and ankle are considered rigid; but with locking mechanisms located at the hip and knee joints, and these parts can move anytime person desires. Therefore, in consequence of any adverse motion, the limb will be protected from harm. Also, in the active orthosis, the system acts from the hip zone and only performs “flexion” and “extension” motions. The HKAFO has two mechanical structures: (1) the gear and T type deflector reducer mechanism to transmit the generated torques of an actuator to the hip joints; and (2) pulley and four-bar mechanism, which is used for transferring the generated torque to the knee joints. With the mechanical system used for the motor to move in both directions, also provided power save, it is being aimed to

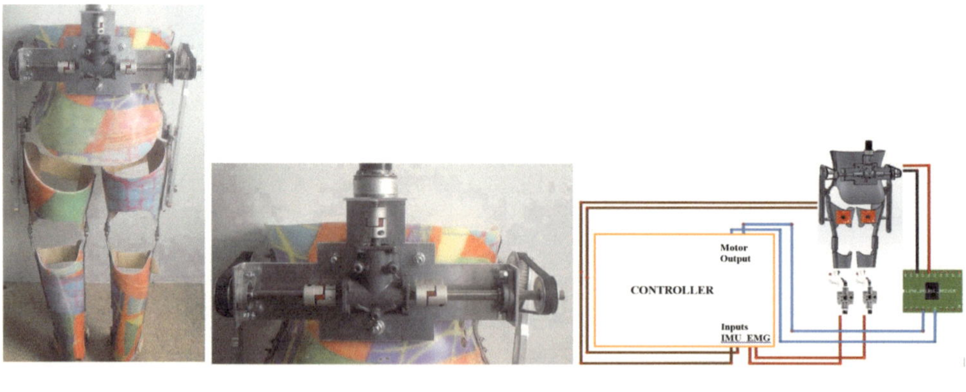

Figure 12.
Hip-knee-ankle-foot-orthosis (HKAFO): (A) system configuration, with T-type deflector reducer; (B) control circuit (online video: [98]).

reduce battery consumption to minimum which was a huge problem in these devices. Illustration of the control circuit is shown in **Figure 12(B)**. The patient's intention to perform a flexion or extension motion is detected by both EMG and accelerometer sensors. In order to determine the last location of the patient after movement, physical feedback is utilized from the mechanical system. Adding the new ankle joint to HKAFOs for real-time virtual limb can also be considered.

The EMG signals may be subject to preprocessing to remove unwanted interference; the most common sources of interference are power line harmonics and motion artifact from electrode movement. As myoelectric signals have a time sequence with a random number of elements, it is not practical for classification. Therefore, the signal sequence should be mapped to feature vectors. Feature vectors of EMG signals are classified to detect which movement produces specific results. Deep neural networks, fuzzy logic, finite state machine and support vector machine, etc. may be adopted as classifiers. In this work, the Finite State Machine (FSM) was chosen as a classifier. The FSM consists of a status set, input, output, event set, and state transition functions. The behavior of each system's state is characterized by a possible system state. Here, the transitions between output states are provided, depending on the input variable and the present state of the system. The EMG signals and the accelerometer data collected from both legs are classified using the FSM method. The result of this classification is used for three different situations for actuator input. These situations are: the patient stops, moves right leg or moves left leg, respectively.

5. Individualized movement choreography

Different users have different health statuses and clinical requirements. VIGOR employs generative deep neural network architecture to create initiative and individualized Tai-Chi movements [26] to benefit users in the most effective way [100–102]. The most *challenging issue* in deep learning enabled choreography is how to balance the training reliability and the creativity of neural network. In this work, we propose the following techniques: (1) visible neural network, which incorporates biomechanics into the neural network, is employed to formulate the generative movement; (2) only mechanical property such as joint/muscle force and moment is used to measure the generative movement; (3) second-order optimizer is used to speed up the training the neural network.

5.1 Tai-Chi choreography based on LSTM-RNN

In this work, Long Short-Term Memory type of RNN (denoted as LSTM) [103, 104] is employed to design individualized Tai-Chi choreography [26]. Human3.6M dataset (high quality 3D joint positions and rotations at 50FPS) and our in-house dataset (acquired by Microsoft Kinect V2, including joints' XYZ and Quaternions, 24-30FPS) are used as the training data. The Tai-Chi movement is created clip by clip (or subsequence by subsequence) according to users' health conditions and their clinical rehabilitation requirements [20].

Figure 13 shows the frame-work of LSTM-based Tai-Chi choreography design. A Tai-Chi movement (or sequence) is partitioned into multiple subsequences (aka a clip or clips). A *seed subsequence*, which can be generated randomly, is fed into the trained model. The output token is regarded as the succeeding subsequence that is fed back into the model for the following subsequence, as a result a creative Tai-Chi sequence can be created clip-by-clip. Four thread visible and hierarchical AutoEncoders [106] are used to reduce problem dimensionality. The resulting individualized Tai-Chi choreography [100–102] is integrated into the VR or AR

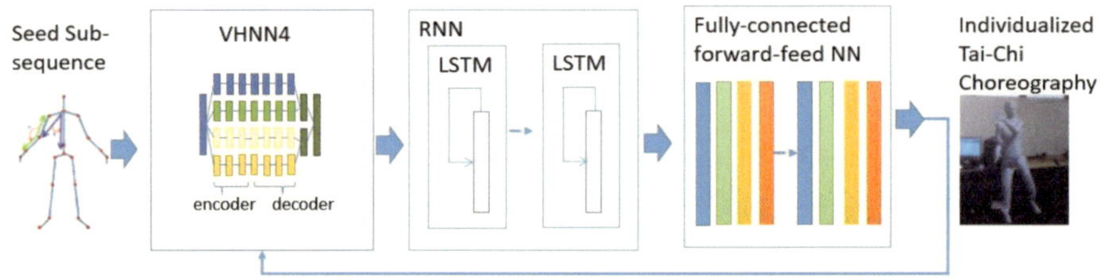

Figure 13.
The pipeline of LSTM-based motion chorepgraphy (online video of LSTM-based Tai-Chi Choreography [88, 105]).

environment [88] from which users can learn. Online video [105] shows a sample Tai-Chi choreography. Compared to other deep learning-enabled choreography projects [107], the proposed method may have faster training speed and be more problem-oriented because (1) the geometric configuration of human anatomy is kept by employing Joint-coordinate systems such as Euler angles. [36, 41], and (2) human biomechanics are preserved by introducing kinetic features [41, 108].

5.2 Movement choreography based on visible GAN

LSTM-based choreography suffers from relatively large accumulated error and lacks a global picture of Tai-Chi choreography. As an effective deep generative model, Generative Adversarial Networks (GANs) learn to model distribution either with or without supervision for high dimensional data (images, texts, audios, etc.), and have been gaining considerable attention in many fields [109–111]. In VIGOR, GANs may be considered to generate novel Tai-Chi movements by simulating a given distribution.

As illustrated in this work, conventional GAN such as DCAN [46], suffers from frequent modal collapse during the training state, particularly on generator side. The discriminator often improves too quickly for the generator to catch up, which is why we need to regulate the learning rates or perform multiple epochs on one of the two networks. To balance the training of generator and discriminator for decent output, this work investigates the following strategies: (1) Application of *Wasserstein distance* to formulate the loss function [46, 112]. (2) Application of *visible neural network* by incorporating the biomechanics theory (inverse dynamics and the transient dynamics simulation of human body [60, 68]) in the formulation of generator and discriminator. The neural network is personalized using boundary and initial conditions of human dynamics.

Figure 14 shows the pipeline of GAN-enabled human movement choreography system. A generator G generates kinematic data out of latent vector, and a discriminator D estimates the probability that a sample came from the training data rather than G. Fed with latent vector, which is randomly generated in the beginning and derived from the transient dynamics simulation of human body thereafter, the generator generates a series of personalized and creative Tai-Chi kinetic subsequence to fool the discriminator. The discriminator is trained to discriminate between "real" Tai-Chi kinetic sub-sequences (from the training set) and "fake" Tai-Chi sub-sequence generated by the generator. Because the generator is fed with deterministic simulated data, an equilibrium of the "adversarial game" between the generator and discriminator can be reached much easily.

In this work, a musculoskeletal biomechanics guided loss function is used to formulate the objective of discriminator:

$$\mathcal{L}(\theta) = L(f(\mathbf{X}, \theta), \mathbf{Y}) + \varrho\mathcal{R}(\theta) + \gamma L_{biomechanics}(f(\mathbf{X}, \theta)) + \eta L_{aesthetics}(f(\mathbf{X}, \theta)) \quad (5)$$

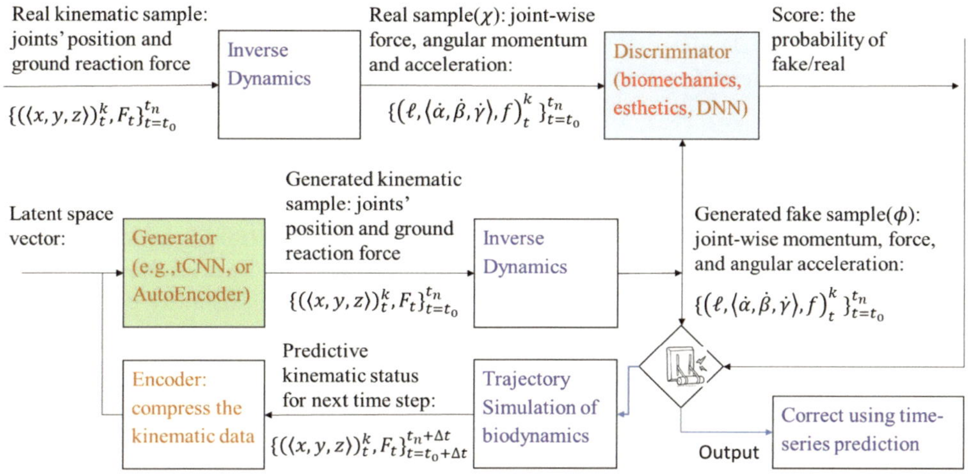

Figure 14.
Movement choreography enabled by visible GAN.

where $\{\mathbf{X}, \mathbf{Y}\}$ indicates labelled training data; $f(\mathbf{X}, \theta)$ is predicting output of neural network; $\theta \in \mathfrak{R}^n$ indicates the parameters (weight and bias) of neural network; $\mathcal{R}(\theta) : \mathfrak{R}^n \to \mathfrak{R}$ is the regularizer, whose importance is controlled by regularization strength $\varrho \in \mathfrak{R}$; same as Eq. (3), $L_{biomechanics}(f(\mathbf{X}, \theta))$ denotes the bio-mechanics violation of choreography with weigh $\gamma \in \mathfrak{R}$; $L_{aesthetics}(f(\mathbf{X}, \theta))$ denotes the violation of athletic elegance violation about the designed choreography with weigh $\eta \in \mathfrak{R}$.

Figure 14 also illustrates that the generated kinetics needs to made temporally consistent according to specific time series prediction models such as ARIMA (Eq. (4)), LSTM, and Fast Fourier Transformation (FFT).

5.3 Polynomial-based Hessian-free Newton–Raphson optimizer

Many deep-learning-enabled applications suffer from training data scarcity. Various strategies have been investigated to overcome this limitation. Besides visible neural network, polynomial-based Hessian-free Newton-Raphson algorithm (poly-HFNR) [69, 113] is proposed to deal with data scarcity issue by speeding up the NN learning efficiency. The superiority of poly-HFNR optimizers includes: (1) A fewer number of training epochs in NN configuration than first-order-convergence optimizers such as stochastic gradient decent (SGD) algorithms; (2) Less computation and storage complexity ($O(N)$ where N is the degree-of-freedom of neural network) than typical implementation of Newton-Raphson based algorithms; (3) Non-convex tolerance; and (4) Circumventing the explicit formulation of the Hessian matrix and the iterative/direct solution to Newton's equations (for optimization) during the training process of the neural network.

Poly-HFNR based on Neumann-series-based (Neumann-poly-HFNR) and poly-HFNR based on generalized least-squared polynomial (GLS-poly-HFNR) [47, 69, 113, 114] have been developed and critically assessed with respect to benchmark problems such as iris-classification, air-foil recognition, simulation of yacht-dynamics, and pima Indian diabetes. Both implementations demonstrate reliable and super-linear convergence performance. The experimental results illustrate that: (1) from the point of view of storage and computation complexity, poly-HFNR is comparable with SGD; (2) from the point of view of convergence performance, poly-HFNR is completely comparable with Quasi-Newton. Our future work will focus on (a) evaluating poly-HFNR on various large-scale benchmark problems; (b) improving the convergence of poly-HFNR from super-linear to quadratic convergence rate; and (c) developing CUDA-version poly-HFNR and then transplanting it into popular deep learning framework such as Pytorch, TensorFlow, and Caffe.

6. Conclusion

This work presents VIGOR system that has a strong potential for broad significance to the physical and psychological health of people with limited mobility. It is expected that VIGOR may (1) produce an affordable and user-friendly platform which promotes regular physical activity via a seamless interaction between the user and the Tai-Chi model/master; (2) cultivate and enhance interdisciplinary research by integrating the expertise of physical therapy, psychology, computer science, electrical engineering, and structural mechanics; and (3) adapt to other movement modalities (e.g, yoga).

The major research elements include: (1) *Seamless real-time 4D human-machine interaction* based on affordable input/output hardware instruments such as Kinect sensor, foot-pressure sensors, actuator, assistive device/exoskeleton, and VR goggle, etc.; (2) *Kinetic movement grading and identification;* (3) *Adaptive virtual limb generation* over VR/AR and assistive device/exoskeketon; and (4) *Individualized movement choreography*(i.e., creative movement design). As the major research contributions of this work, visible and hierarchical neural network (VHNN) architecture is proposed to recognize and predict human kinetics efficiently; and a polynomial-based, Newton-Raphson algorithm is proposed for efficient optimization. Both techniques play significant roles in small-data problems.

As part of our future work, the clinical effect of VIGOR system will be assessed. Specifically, we plan to evaluate both the user-experience and the feasibility of VIGOR by conducting a few of phases of a human subject study with healthy and mobility-limited adult human subjects. In every phase, subjects will be surveyed and interviewed following exposure to VIGOR. The clinical data will be analyzed using Auto-Regressive Integrated Moving Average (ARIMA) model [44].

Acknowledgements

This work was jointly sponsored by National Science Foundation (NSF) 1924278, 1761839 and 1647175.

Author details

Yu Liang*, Dalei Wu, Dakila Ledesma, Zibin Guo, Erkan Kaplanoglu and Anthony Skjellum
University of Tennessee at Chattanooga, USA

*Address all correspondence to: yu-liang@utc.edu

References

[1] Marini, I., and Stebnicki, M. A. The Psychological and Social Impact of Illness and Disability, 6th Ed. Springer publishing, 2012.

[2] [report] physical inactivity among adults 50 years and older - united states, 2014. Morbidity and Mortality Weekly Report 2016 65, 36 (2016).

[3] Kelley, G., Kelley, K., Hootman, J., and Jones, D. Effects of community-deliverable exercise on pain and physical function in adults with arthritis and other rheumatic diseases: a meta-analysis. Arthritis Care Res. 63, 1 (2011), 79–93.

[4] Fasko, D. Tai chi chuan and physical and psychological health: a review. Journal of American Kinesiotherapy Association 55 (2001), 4–12.

[5] Cho, K. Effect of tai chi on depressive symptoms amongst chinese older patients with major depression: the role of social support. Medicine and Sport Science 52 (2008), 146–154.

[6] Taylor-Piliae, R., and Haskell, W. Tai chi exercise and stroke rehabilitation. Topics in Stroke Rehabilitation 14 (2007), 9–22.

[7] Cheung, S., Tsai, E., Fung, L., and Ng, J. Physical benefits of tai chi chuan for individuals with lower-limb disabilities. Occupational Therapy International 14 (2007), 1–10.

[8] Wang, C., Schmid, C., and Rones, R. A randomized trial of tai chi for fibromyalgia. New England Journal of Medicine 363 (2010), 743–754.

[9] Taggart, H., Arslanian, C., Bae, S., and Singh, K. Effects of t'ai chi exercise on fibromyalgia symptoms and health-related quality of life. Orthopedic Nursing 22 (2003), 353–360.

[10] Klein, P., and Adams, W. Cardiopulmonary physiotherapeutic application of tai ji. Journal of Cardiopulmonary Physical Therapy 15 (2004), 5–11.

[11] Hong, Y., Li, J., and Robinson, P. Balance control, flexibility, and cardiorespiratory fitness among older tai chi practitioners. British Journal of Sports Medicine 34 (2000), 29–34.

[12] Taylor, E., and Taylor-Piliae, R. The effects of tai chi on physical and psychosocial function among persons with multiple sclerosis: A systematic review. Complementary Therapies in Medicine 31 (2017), 100–108.

[13] Song, R., Grabowska, W., Park, M., Osypiuk, K., Hausdorff, J., Fox, M., Sudarsky, L., Macklin, E., and Wayne, P. The impact of tai chi and qigong mind-body exercises on moor and non-motor function abd quality of life in parkinson's disease: A systematic review and meta-analysis. Parkinsonism and Related Disordersa 41 (2017), 3–13.

[14] McGibbon, C., David, E., Wolf, S., and Wayne, P. Tai chi and vestibular rehabilitation effects on gaze and whole-body stability. Journal of Vestibular Research 14 (2004), 467–478.

[15] Wang, C., Collet, J., and Lau, J. The effect of tai chi on health outcomes in patients with chronic conditions: a systematic review. Archives of Internal Medicine 164 (2004), 493–501.

[16] Wang, C., Bannuru, R., Ramel, J., Kupelnic, B., Scott, T., and Schmid, C. Tai chi on psychological well-being: systematic review and meta-analysis. J. of Complementary Alternative Med. 10, 23 (2010), 1–16.

[17] [report] centers for disease control and prevention. prevalence of self-reported physically active adults –

united states, 2007. Morbidity and Mortality Weekly Report 2008 57, 48 (2008), 1297–1300.

[18] F., S., and E., P. Counteracting physical inactivity during the covid-19 pandemic: Evidence-based recommendations for home-based exercise. Int J Environ Res Public Health 17, 11 (6 2020), 3909.

[19] Asay, G., Roy, K., Lang, J., Payne, R., and Howard, D. Absenteeism and employer costs associated with chronic diseases and health risk factors in the us workforce. Prev Chronic Dis. 13, 150503 (2016).

[20] Liang, Y., Wu, D., Dakila, D., Davis, C., Slaughter, R., and Guo, Z. B. Virtual taiji system, a smart-connected modality for rehabilitation. In The Third IEEE/ACM Conference on Connected Health: Applications, Systems, and System Technologies (Washington, D.C., Sept. 26–28 2018).

[21] Bond, D., Lyle, R., Tappe, M., Seehafer, R., and D'Zurilla, T. Moderate aerobic exercise, tai chi, and social problem-solving ability in relation to psychological stress. International Journal of Stress Management 9 (2002), 329–343.

[22] Liang, Y., Ledesma, D., and Wu, D. [online] vtcs: virtuality coaching based on unity 3d. https://www.youtube.com/watch?v=OQySt2i8dzo&feature=youtu.be. Cited May 8, 2018.

[23] Patel, S., Park, H., Bonato, P., Chan, L., and Rodgers, M. A review of wearable sensors and systems with application in rehabilitation. Journal of NeuroEngineering and Rehabilitation (2012), 9:21.

[24] Chen, K., Chen, P., Liu, K., and Chan, C. Wearable sensor-based rehabilitation exercise assessment for knee osteoarthritis. Sensors 15 (2015), 4193–4211.

[25] Sprint, G., Cook, D., Weeks, D., Dahmen, J., and Fleur, A. Analyzing sensor-based time series data to track changes in physical activity during inpatient rehabilitation. Sensors 17, 10 (2017).

[26] Guo, Z. Thirteen postures of wheelchair taijiquan (tai chi): Wheelchair use as an instrument of empowerment. Journal of Technology and Innovation - Proceedings of the National Academy of Inventors 13, 4 (2012), 267–279.

[27] Guo, Z. A short survey of the development of traditional chinese medicine in china. Journal of Education about Asia 15, 2 (2000), 46–49.

[28] Taylor-Piliae, R., Haskell, W., Waters, C., and Froelicher, E. Change in perceived psychosocial status following a 12-week tai chi exercise programme. Journal of Advanced Nursing 54 (2006), 313–329.

[29] Silverman, A., and Neptune, R. Muscle and prosthesis contributions to amputee walking mechanics: a modeling study. Journal of Biomechanics 45, 13 (2012), 2271–2278.

[30] Pickle, N., Wilken, J., Whitehead, J. A., and Silverman, A. Whole-body angular momentum during sloped walking using passive and powered lower-limb prostheses. Journal of Biomechanics, 14 (2016), 3397–3406.

[31] Silverman, A.K. J.M. Wilken, E. S., and Neptune, R. Whole-body angular momentum during incline and decline walking. Journal of Biomechanics, 6 (2012), 965–971.

[32] Hegarty, A.K., Kurz, M., Stuberg, W., and Silverman, A. Strength training effects on muscle forces and contributions to whole body movement in cerebral palsy. Journal of Motor Behavior, 5 (2019), 496–510.

[33] Alkan, B., Fidan, F., Tosun, A., and Ardicoglu, O. Quality of life and self-reported disability in patients with knee osteoarthritis. Mod Rheumatol 24, 1 (Jan 2014), 166–171.

[34] Wang, C., Schmid, C., Iversen, M., Harvey, W., Fielding, R., Driban, J., Price, L., Wong, J., Reid, K., Rones, R., and McAlindon, T. Comparative effectiveness of tai chi versus physical therapy for knee osteoarthritis. Ann Intern Med 165, 2 (July 19 2016), 77–86.

[35] Ledesma, D., Ledesma, D., Slaughter, R., Wu, D., Guo, Z., and Liang, Y. Kinetic gesture recognition and choreography. In IEEE BigDataService 2018 (Bamberg, Germany, March 26–29 2018).

[36] Davis, C., Ledesma, D., Slaughter, R., Wu, D., Guo, Z., and Liang, Y. Kinetic data processing for gesture recognition. In IEEE BigDataService 2018 (Bamberg, Germany, March 26–29 2018).

[37] Bengio, Y. Learning deep architectures for ai. fundamental Trends Machine Learning 2, 1 (January 2009), 1–127.

[38] Steffen, T., and TA, T. H. Age- and gender-related test performance in community-dwelling elderly people: Six-minute walk test, berg balance scale, timed up & go test, and gait speeds. Physical Therapy 82, 2 (2002), 128–137.

[39] Tiwana, M., Redmond, S., and Lovell, N. A review of tactile sensing technologies with applications in biomedical engineering. Sensors and Actuators A: Physical 179 (2012), 17–31.

[40] Liang, Y., Wu, D., Huston, D., Liu, G. R., Li, Y., Gao, C., and Ma, J. Chapter 12: Civil Infrastructure Serviceability Evaluation Based on Big Data. Springer Publishing, June 2018.

[41] Liang, Y., Guo, Z. B., Wu, D. L., Fell, N., and Clark, A. Virtual taiji system - an innovative modality for rehabilitation. In Annual BSEC Conference at Oak Ridge National Laboratory Collaborative Biomedical Innovations (08/25–27 2015).

[42] Rai, R., and Sahu, C. K. Driven by data or derived through physics? a review of hybrid physics guided machine learning techniques with cyber-physical system (cps) focus. IEEE Access 8 (2020), 71050–71073.

[43] Zhang, Z., and Sun, C. Structural damage identification via physics-guided machine learning: a methodology integrating pattern recognition with finite element model updating. Structural Health Monitoring 0, 0 (0), 1475921720927488.

[44] Ho, S. L., and Xie, M. The use of arima models for reliability forecasting and analysis. Comput. Ind. Eng. 35, 1–2 (Oct. 1998), 213–216.

[45] Ferris, D. P., Sawicki, G. S., and Domingo, A. Powered lower limb orthoses for gait rehabilitation. Topics in spinal cord injury rehabilitation 11, 2 (2005), 34–49.

[46] Goodfellow, I., Bengio, Y., and Courville, A. Deep Learning. MIT Press, 2016.

[47] Liang, Y., and Haney, R. A polynomial-based hessian-free-newton-raphson optimizer for the training of neural network. arXiv.org (2018), 1–20.

[48] Farebrother, R. W., Grob, J., and Troschke, S.-O. Matrix representation of quaternions. Linear Algebra and its Applications 362 (2003), 251–255.

[49] ES, G., and WJ, S. A joint coordinate system for the clinical description of three-dimensional motions: application to the knee. J Biomech Eng. 105, 2 (May 1983), 136–144.

[50] Shoemake, K. Animating rotation with quaternion curve. SIGGRAPH '85

proceedings, Computer Graphics 19, 3 (July 22–26 1985), 245–255.

[51] S.Hawran, and Sorenson, F. B. The use of long leg calipers for paraplegic patients: a follow up study of patients discharged. Spinal Cord (1996), 666–668.

[52] Lee, E. Cyber physical systems: Design challenges. In Proc. of IEEE International Symposium on Object Oriented Real-time Distributed Computing (ISORC) (2008).

[53] Sha, L., Gopalakrishnan, S., Liu, X., and Wang, Q. Cyber-physical systems: A new frontier. In Proc. of IEEE International Conference on Sensor Networks, Ubiquitous and Trustworthy Computing (2008).

[54] Hu, Y., Patel, M., Sabella, D., Sprecher, N., and Young, V. Mobile edge computing a key technology towards 5g. European Telecommunications Standards Institute (ETSI) White Paper (September 2015).

[55] Mkinen, O. Streaming at the edge: Local service concepts utilizing mobile edge computing. In The 9th International Conference on Next Generation Mobile Applications, Services and Technologies (2015).

[56] Ledesma, D., Baker, W., and Liang, Y. [online] vtcs: Deployment of vtcs over commodity hardware. https://youtu.be/_bB8K627JZk. cite July 04, 2018.

[57] Bulling, A., Blanke, U., and Schiele, B. A tutorial on human activity recognition using body-worn inertial sensors. ACM Computing Surveys 46, 3 (2014), 1–33.

[58] Ding, H., Trajcevski, G., Scheuermann, P., Wang, X., and Keogh, E. Querying and mining of time series data: Experimental comparison of representations and distance measures. Proceedings of the VLDB Endowment 1, 2 (2008), 1542–1552.

[59] Lin, J., Williamson, S., Borne, K., and DeBarr, D. Pattern Recognition in Time Series. Taylor & Francis Group, 2012.

[60] Pizzolato, C., Reggiani, M., Modenese, L., and Lloyd, D. G. Real-time inverse kinematics and inverse dynamics for lower limb applications using opensim. Computer Methods in Biomechanics and Biomedical Engineering 20, 4 (2017), 436–445. PMID: 27723992.

[61] Alharbi, N., Liang, Y., and Wu, D. Extended-kalman-filter preprocessing technique for gesture recognition. In 2nd IEEE/ACM CHASE (Philadelphia, USA, July 17–19 2017).

[62] Liang, Y., Ledesma, D., Davis, C., Slaughter, R., and Wu, D. [online] vtcs: preprocessed and raw kinematic data (front view). https://www.youtube.com/watch?v=KFBV_EBTEQw. Cited March 2, 2018.

[63] Liang, Y., Ledesma, D., Davis, C., Slaughter, R., and Wu, D. [online] vtcs: preprocessed and raw kinematic data (front and back view). https://youtu.be/Ee31SdhXxXc. Cited March 2, 2018.

[64] Ambrosio, J., and Kecskemethy, a. Multibody dynamics of biomechanical models for human motion via optimization. Multibody Dynamics: Computational Method and Application, J.C. Garcia Orden et al. (Eds) 6 (2007), 245–272.

[65] Ehsani, H., Rostami, M., and Gudarzi, M. A general-purpose framework to simulate musculoskeletal system of human body: using a motion tracking approach. Computer Methods in Biomechanics and Biomedical Engineering 19, 3 (2016), 306–319. PMID: 25761607.

[66] Eich-Soellner, E., and Führer, C. Numerical Methods in Multibody Dynamics. Teubner, Stuttgart, 2008.

[67] Moreira, P., Lugrís, U., Cuadrado, J., and Flores, P. Biomechanical models for human gait analyses using inverse dynamics formulation. Sociedade Portuguesa de Biomecânica, 2013.

[68] Ezati, M., Ghannadi, B., and McPhee, J. A review of simulation methods for human movement dynamics with emphasis on gait. Multibody System Dynamics (May 2019).

[69] Liang, Y., Szularz, M., and Yang, L. T. Finite-element-wise domain decomposition iterative solvers based on polynomial preconditioning. Mathematical and Computer Modeling 58, 1–2 (July 2013), 421–437.

[70] Wittenburg, J. Dynamics of Multibody Systems. Berlin, Springer, 2008.

[71] Liang, Y., Wu, D., Dakila, D., Davis, C., Slaughter, R., and Guo, Z. B. Virtual tai-chi system, a smart connected modality for rehabilitation. Elsevier: Smart Health 9–10 (12 2018), 232–249.

[72] Kalman, R. A new approach to linear filtering and prediction problems. Journal of Basic Engineering 80 (1960), 35.

[73] Einicke, G. Smoothing, Filtering and Prediction: Estimating the Past, Present and Future. Rijeka, Croatia: Intech, 2012.

[74] Zarchan, P., and Musoff, H. Fundamentals of Kalman Filtering: A Practical Approach. American Institute of Aeronautics and Astronautics, Incorporated, 2000.

[75] Sperduti, A., and Starita, A. Supervised neural networks for the classification of structures. IEEE Transactions on Neural Networks 8, 3 (May 1995), 714–735.

[76] Richman, J., and Moorman, J. Physiological time-series analysis using approximate entropy and sample entropy. American Journal of Physiological Heart Circ Physiol. 278, 6 (Jun. 2000), H2039–H2049.

[77] Hansen, C., Wei, Q., Shieh, J., Fourcade, P., Isableu, B., and Majed, L. Sample entropy, univariate, and multivariate multi-scale entropy in comparison with classical postural sway parameters in young healthy adults. Front. Hum. Neuroscience 11 (2017), 206–217.

[78] Duda, R. O., Hart, P. E., and Stork, D. G. Pattern Classification (2nd Edition). Wiley-Interscience, 2000.

[79] Keogh, E. Data Mining and Machine Learning in Time Series Databases. Springer, 2004.

[80] Yang, K., and Shahaby, C. An efficient k-nearest neighbor search for multivariate time series. Information and Computation 205 (2007), 65–98.

[81] Eads, D., Hill, D., Davis, S., Perkins, S., Ma, J., Porter, R., and Theiler, J. Genetic algorithms and support vector machines for time series classification. Proc. SPIE 4787 (July 2002), 74–85.

[82] Schlkopf, B., and Smola, A. J. Learning with Kernels: Support Vector Machines, Regularization, Optimization, and Beyond (Adaptive Computation and Machine Learning). The MIT Press, 2001.

[83] Geurts, P. Pattern extraction for time series classification. In In proceedings of the 5th European Conference on Principles of Data Mining and Knowledge Discovery (Freiburg, Germany, 2001), pp. 115–127.

[84] Han, J., and Kamber, M. Data Mining: Concepts and Techniques. Morgan Kaufmann Publishers Inc., San Francisco, CA, USA., 2000.

[85] Chen, C., Jafari, R., and Kehtarnavaz, N. [online] utd-mhad:

Benchmark kinect data set. http://www.utdallas.edu/~kehtar/UTD-MHAD.html. Cited 2015.

[86] LU XiA. [online] kinect: View invariant human action recognition using histograms of 3d joints. http://cvrc.ece.utexas.edu/KinectDatasets/HOJ3D.html. Cited 2017.

[87] Liang, Y., Ledesma, D., Davis, C., Slaughter, R., and Wu, D. [online] scprs: coaching through visual and verbal instruction. https://www.youtube.com/watch?v=ickqTwBjcUs. Cited August 17, 2016.

[88] Liang, Y., Ledesma, D., and Wu, D. [online] vtcs: individualized virtual tai-chi master in augmented reality environment. https://www.youtube.com/watch?v=JCPD8jloo64&feature=youtu.be. Cited May 20, 2018.

[89] Ledesma, D., Liang, Y., and Wu, D. Adaptive generation of phantom limbs using visible hierarchical autoencoders. CoRR abs/1910.01191 (2019).

[90] Ledesma, D., and Liang, Y. [online] vtcs: Construct phantom legs according to arms' movement using varius autoencoder strategies. https://youtu.be/ZmTobUjRX64. cite November 08, 2018.

[91] Murphy, A. C., Muldoon, S. F., Baker, D., Lastowka, A., Bennett, B., Yang, M., and Bassett, D. S. Structure, function, and control of the human musculoskeletal network. plos biology.

[92] Ledesma, D., and Liang, Y. [online] playlist of phantom legs induced by moving arms. https://www.youtube.com/playlist?list=PL8VO3nxhbh0IngDo5ij0PkKxK5uFbtXE0. Cite December 08, 2018.

[93] Ledesma, D., and Liang, Y. [online] vtcs: Construct phantom legs according to arms' movement using 7-layer mlp. https://youtu.be/BFW3JVI0dKM. cite December 08, 2018.

[94] Ledesma, D., and Liang, Y. [online] vtcs: Construct phantom legs according to arms' movement using autoencoder. https://youtu.be/1aHJQyST9k0. cite December 08, 2018.

[95] Ledesma, D., and Liang, Y. [online] vtcs: Construct phantom legs according to arms' movement using two-thead vhnn autoencoder. https://youtu.be/pVtzw0dJduA. cite December 08, 2018.

[96] Ledesma, D., and Liang, Y. [online] vtcs: Construct phantom legs according to arms' movement using four-thead vhnn autoencoder. https://youtu.be/dGPm4z7vibI. cite December 08, 2018.

[97] Ulkir, O., Akgun, G., and Kaplanoglu, E. Mechanical design and analysis of a pneumatic ankle foot orthosis. 2018 Electric Electronics, Computer Science, Biomedical Engineering' Meeting (EBBT) (2018), 1–4.

[98] Kaplanoglu, E. [online] active hip-knee-ankle-foot orthosis (a-hkafo). https://www.youtube.com/watch?v=JbFSDunV8Js. Cite September 20, 2019.

[99] Webster, J. B., and Murphy, D. P. Atlas of Orthoses and Assistive Devices (Fifth Edition). 2019.

[100] Berman, A., and James, V. Kinetic imaginations: Exploring the possibilities of combining ai and dance. In Proceedings of the Twenty-Fourth International Joint Conference on Artificial Intelligence (IJCAI 2015) (Buenos Aires, Argentina, 25–31 July 2015), pp. 2431–2437.

[101] Briot, J.-P., Hadjeres, G., and Pachet, F. Deep learning techniques for music generation – a survey. arXiv:1709.01620 (2018), 1–108.

[102] Donahue, C., Lipton, Z. C., and McAuley, J. Dance dance convolution. CoRR abs/1703.06891 (2017).

[103] Hammer, B. Learning with Recurrent Neural Networks. Springer, October 2007.

[104] Hochreiter, S., and Schmidhuber, J. Long short-term memory. Neural Computation 9, 8 (1997), 1735–1780.

[105] Liang, Y., and Ledesma, D. [online] vtcs: Tai-chi choreography derived from lstm-rnn. https://youtu.be/phcncKvq4hQ. cite June 18, 2018.

[106] Géron, A. Hands-On Machine Learning with Scikit-Learn and TensorFlow. O'Reilly, 2017.

[107] Crnkovic-Friis, L., and Crnkovic-Friis, L. Generative choreography using deep learning. ICCC (2016).

[108] Yuan, X., Kong, L., Feng, D., and Wei, Z. Automatic feature point detection and tracking of human action in time-of-flight videos. IEEE/CAA Journal of Automatica Sinica 4, 4 (Oct. 2017), 677–685.

[109] Goodfellow, I., Pouget-Abadie, J., Mirza, M., Xü, B., Warde-Farley, D., Ozair, S., Courville, A., and Bengio, Y. Generative adversarial nets. In Proc. of Advances in Neural Information Processing Systems (2014).

[110] Elgammal, A., Liu, B., Elhoseiny, M., and Mazzone, M. Can: Creative adversarial networks generating "art" by learning about styles and deviating from style norms. arXiv:1706.07068 6 (2017), 1–22.

[111] Hong, Y., Hwang, U., Yoo, J., and Yoon, S. How generative adversarial networks and their variants work: An overview of gan. arXiv:1711.05914v7, July 2018.

[112] Endres, D. M., and Schindelin, J. E. A new metric for probability distributions. IEEE Transactions on Information Theory 49, 7 (July 2003), 1858–1860.

[113] Liang, Y., Shi, Z., and Chung, P. A hessian-free newton-raphson method for the configuration of physics systems featured by numerically asymmetric force field. Mathematical and Computer Simulation (February 2017), 1–23.

[114] Liang, Y., Weston, J., and Szularz, M. Generalized least-squares polynomial preconditioners for symmetric indefinite linear equations. Parallel computing (Impact Factor: 1.693) 28, 2 (2002), 323–341.